GOOD LIVING WITH
Rheumatoid Arthritis

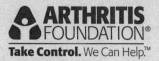

Published by:
The Arthritis Foundation
1330 West Peachtree Street, NW, Suite 100
Atlanta, GA 30309

Library of Congress Card Catalog Number: 2004107995

ISBN: 0-912423-50-1

The Arthritis Foundation is proud to
be a participating organization in
the Bone and Joint Decade.

Participating Organization

Bone
and Joint
DECADE
—— 2002 - USA - 2011 ——

The mission of the Arthritis Foundation
is to improve lives through leadership
in the prevention, control and cure of
arthritis and related diseases.

Table of Contents

PART ONE: Learn All You Can

Chapter 1. Understanding Arthritis: Cleaning Up Myths and
Exploring Treatment Approaches

Chapter 2. Understanding Rheumatoid Arthritis:
A Chronic, Complex Disease

Chapter 3. Diagnosing Rheumatoid Arthritis:
Your Medical History and Physical Examination

PART THREE: DEVELOP A GOOD LIVING LIFESTYLE

FOREWORD

To make comparisons among the 100 or more forms of arthritis is difficult, impossible really. Each touches the lives of those affected in personal and often profound ways.

By whatever standard one might choose, however, rheumatoid arthritis ranks high as one of the most serious forms of arthritis. Although rheumatoid arthritis can begin at any age including childhood, women between ages 40 and 50 are most commonly affected. Joint pain and limitations become a daily experience and interfere with essentially all activities – those essential for simply making it through the day as well as those for pleasure. Moreover, for most people, the arthritis becomes chronic and persists for their lifetime. Over years, rheumatoid arthritis damages and deforms joints, hands, and wrists, further limiting a person's ability to use them.

For many people with rheumatoid arthritis, the uncertainty of knowing what the future holds and the frustration of scant symptom relief pose major challenges. Fortunately, the situation is changing rapidly. In the past decade alone, researchers have made remarkable progress in the scientific understanding of rheumatoid arthritis, providing important clues that have already resulted in newer, more effective drugs. Ongoing research will continue to teach us about the disease. In fact, curing or even preventing rheumatoid arthritis seems a real and distinct possibility.

The Arthritis Foundation believes that the actions of people with rheumatoid arthritis play an important role in determining the outcome of the disease and its impact on their lives. Education, self-help and personal responsibility are tools of empowerment – keys to working effectively with physicians to achieve control of rheumatoid arthritis. This book, *Good Living With Rheumatoid Arthritis*, is a resource guide for people with rheumatoid arthritis, their families and loved ones, offering help in understanding the disease and improving their lives.

John H. Klippel, MD
President and Chief Executive Officer
Arthritis Foundation, Atlanta, GA

ACKNOWLEDGMENTS

Good Living With Rheumatoid Arthritis is written for people who have rheumatoid arthritis, as well as for their friends, family and loved ones. Bringing this book to completion was a team effort, including the contributions of physicians, health-care professionals, Arthritis Foundation staff and volunteers, writers, editors, designers.

Special acknowledgments should go to the medical editor of the original edition of this book, Theodore Pincus, MD, Professor of Medicine at Vanderbilt University School of Medicine, as well as to his co-editor, Cynthia M. Kahn. The chief medical reviewer of the book is John H. Klippel, MD, President and Chief Executive Officer of the Arthritis Foundation.

The panel that reviewed the book includes rheumatologists Joan Bathon, MD, Johns Hopkins Bayview Medical Center, Division of Rheumatology, Baltimore, MD; Marcy Bolster, MD, Medical University of South Carolina, Division of Rheumatology and Immunology, Charleston, SC; Doyt L. Conn, MD, Emory University School of Medicine and Grady Health System, Division of Rheumatology/Immunology, Atlanta, Ga.; and Mary Corr, MD, University of California, San Diego, School of Medicine. In addition, Jennifer Lewis, an Arthritis Foundation volunteer who also has rheumatoid arthritis, reviewed the original edition of this book for accuracy from the patient's perspective. Additional thanks go to Gretchen Henkel, who served as a writer on the early stages of the book's development. Dorothy Foltz-Gray edited this edition.

The editorial director of this edition is Bethany Afshar. The art director of the book is Tracie Bullis.

Introduction

INTRODUCTION

The most important person managing your rheumatoid arthritis (RA) is you. That's why the Arthritis Foundation organized this book around the five most significant habits you can develop to manage your disease. We're convinced that if you follow the advice the book offers, you can deal with your RA more effectively.

The first step for anyone in managing a medical problem is to learn as much as possible about their disease. The more you know about the physical and mental landscape of rheumatoid arthritis, its causes and treatments, the better equipped you will be to handle the changes it brings to your life. Now more than ever before, medical research is yielding new information about both conventional and alternative therapies for treating the disease's many symptoms.

As important as your education is the relationship you form with the doctors, nurses and specialists who will work with you to manage the disease. Doctors vary as much as patients do, and finding one whom you feel confident about and comfortable with will affect the quality of your care. Understanding what your doctor needs and expects will also affect your treatment, psychologically and physically.

No matter what your doctor recommends, you're the only person who can implement the therapies you decide on together. No quick fix exists for RA. Your surest route to feeling better depends on early and aggressive treatment combined with the daily good living habits you develop. Research has proven that a healthy diet, regular exercise and satisfying personal relationships are all essential features of well-being. None of those things, together or separately, can make arthritis disappear, but each is an important part of staying and feeling well.

Although you will have days when you feel that RA is the boss, you can control many of the choices that affect how you feel. Learning to set goals, solve problems and prioritize how you spend your energy will help you deal with the disease. The more you learn about ways to alter the aspects of your life that work against your disease, the better you will feel.

Depression, grief and stress can all accompany rheumatoid arthritis. Accepting, understanding and working through those tough emotions is an important habit, as crucial as daily exercise or self-education. The book will begin to show you how to deal with RA's many challenges.

Unfortunately, there is no cure for rheumatoid arthritis and finding relief isn't always as quick as we'd like. But with education, aggressive treatment and persistence, you can achieve good living with this disease. With a commitment to help yourself, you can feel better. That option lies within your power. Consider this book a resource and guide in the journey to a better life.

PART ONE

Learn All You Can

Chapter 1

Understanding Arthritis:
Clearing Up Myths and Exploring Treatment Approaches

The goal of this book is to give you strategies and information that can help you achieve good living with rheumatoid arthritis. Before we get started, though, it's necessary to take a step back and look at the big picture. This chapter may be used as a building block for understanding the complex condition known as rheumatoid arthritis.

Arthritis is a term derived from the Greek words "arth" (meaning joint) and "itis" (meaning inflammation). Its literal meaning is "joint inflammation." However, the word *arthritis* is often used to refer to any of the more than 100 conditions that cause pain in the joints and tissues surrounding them, such as muscles and tendons (which connect muscles to bone). The conditions may be called *forms of arthritis, musculoskeletal conditions* or *rheumatic diseases*. In many sources – including this book – the terms are used interchangeably.

The physicians who specialize in diagnosing and treating arthritis and related rheumatic diseases are called *rheumatologists*. People who experience symptoms such as joint pain or swelling may not initially seek the care of a rheumatologist because they may not know that they should. They may make an appointment with their regular, primary-care physician, such as an internist or family physician. Or they may schedule an appointment with an orthopaedist, a doctor who specializes in treating bone disorders and ailments. These physicians can refer patients to a rheumatologist if necessary for diagnosis or treatment. Children can also have forms of arthritis, including juvenile rheumatoid arthritis. These children should seek diagnosis and treatment from a pediatric rheumatologist if at all possible. These physicians specialize in the treatment of juvenile rheumatic diseases in children and adolescents.

Arthritis Myths

Arthritis has been recognized for thousands of years. Even prehistoric skeletal remains of humans show signs of arthritis. Unfortunately, the myths about arthritis have been around for almost as long. We will try to debunk some of these myths about arthritis and provide key definitions along the way.

Myth #1: Arthritis Is Just Aches and Pains

One common myth is that arthritis is just another name for the aches and pains we get as we get older. Although arthritis does become more common as people age, the condition may begin at any age, including childhood. And some elderly people never develop arthritis. Many forms of arthritis or musculoskeletal conditions are self-limited and get better without specific treatment. Others, such as rheumatoid arthritis, may be quite serious and may affect the body's internal organs as well as the joints.

Major Myths

- Arthritis is just another name for joint aches and pains associated with aging.

- Arthritis isn't really a serious health problem.

- Not much can be done to help people with arthritis.

A simple way to organize arthritis-related conditions is to group them into categories based on whether they affect only one joint or area of the body (localized conditions) or many joints and organs over the entire body (generalized conditions), as shown in the box. Localized conditions include two subgroups. The first subgroup includes conditions that affect the soft tissues surrounding joints and bones but do not affect the structure of joints or bones directly. These are known as soft-tissue, localized conditions, and include tendinitis and bursitis. The second subgroup includes conditions that affect one or a few joints, such as a single knee or hip. A common example of this second subgroup is osteoarthritis of a single joint, although osteoarthritis often affects more than one joint.

Likewise, generalized conditions can be divided into two subgroups. The first subgroup – widespread muscle and soft tissue discomfort without evidence of swelling or inflammation – includes a common condition called *fibromyalgia.* Conditions in this subgroup are not associated with damage to the structure of the joints. The second subgroup includes conditions in which inflammation affects the entire body, such as rheumatoid arthritis. Other conditions in this subgroup include gout, ankylosing spondylitis and psoriatic arthritis, generalized conditions of inflammation throughout the body in which joint pain is the major symptom. Other generalized inflammatory conditions include polymyositis, which primarily affects muscles; systemic lupus erythematosus (lupus), which may affect the skin, kidney or other organs; and vasculitis, which may affect any organ.

These four groups of musculoskeletal conditions are not mutually exclusive, and a person may have more than one type of rheumatic disease. For example, people with rheumatoid arthritis may experience tendinitis, bursitis and fibromyalgia more commonly than people in the general population. In addition, when joints become badly damaged as a result of the chronic inflammation of rheumatoid arthritis, they are called *end stage.* At this point, the joints may look similar to those that have reached end stage in people with osteoarthritis, even though the destruction was caused by different mechanisms.

Arthritis-Related Conditions

Localized conditions (affecting one joint or one area of the body)

- Soft tissue localized conditions (bursitis or tendinitis, for example)

- Conditions that affect one or a few joints (such as osteoarthritis)

Generalized conditions (affecting many joints or areas of the body)

- Widespread muscle/soft tissue conditions without inflammation (such as fibromyalgia)

- Inflammatory conditions usually involving joints (psoriatic arthritis, gout, vasculitis and ankylosing spondylitis)

Myth #2: Arthritis Isn't Really a Serious Health Problem

Arthritis and related rheumatic diseases, as well as chronic joint symptoms, are the most common chronic health conditions in the population, affecting about 70 million Americans. The conditions become more common among older people. Even in people under age 65, arthritis is the leading cause of work disability. For example, fewer than 50 percent of rheumatoid arthritis patients younger than 65 who are working at the onset of the disease are working 10 years later.

In addition, the impact of arthritis on society is substantial. According to the Centers for Disease Control and Prevention, costs associated with arthritis amount to approximately $86 billion annually, an economic impact on par with a moderate recession. The costs of arthritis fall into three groups: direct, indirect and intangible. Direct medical costs, such as physician (and other health professional) fees, charges for laboratory tests and X-rays, drugs, assistive devices, surgeries and other costs, are the most obvious. However, a substantial part of the economic burden is indirect costs such as lost wages due to work disability. In addition, people experience intangible costs, such as the need for a spouse or relative to take time off from work to take a patient to

a caregiver or for medical care, or to remodel a home to meet the physical needs of a person with arthritis.

Myth #3: Not Much Can Be Done to Alleviate the Pain and Disability of Arthritis

Unfortunately, there are no cures for most chronic rheumatic conditions. You may think that little can be done to help your arthritis. This is not true: Almost everyone with arthritis can lessen pain and loss of function. Furthermore, the disease process that may lead to joint destruction can be controlled effectively in most people – particularly those with rheumatoid arthritis. In fact, more can be done today to ease the pain of arthritis and to slow joint destruction than ever before. The first step to take is to see a qualified doctor and get an accurate diagnosis.

Many people with serious types of arthritis, which were severely disabling as recently as a generation ago, are now leading full and productive lives thanks in part to many developments including new drugs and treatments, exercise programs, surgeries and self-management. Your future, as a person with arthritis, is full of possibilities that were only a dream 25 years ago.

One of the most exciting changes in recent years has been the growing understanding that the patient has an important role to play in the management of his or her arthritis. The change in emphasis is sometimes referred to as a *biopsychosocial model of disease management* to distinguish it from the traditional biomedical model in which disease outcomes are thought to be determined by the actions of health professionals. Of course, the wonderful advances in drugs, surgeries and other medical treatments are an important component of a biopsychosocial model of disease management. But this model also incorporates the key contribution of patients, families and support networks to

the outcome. In the second part of this chapter, we will focus on this model, which lays the groundwork for many of the ideas expressed in this book.

The Biopsychosocial Model for Arthritis Care

The biomedical model of medical care evolved in the late 19th and early 20th century, based on the idea of identifying a single cause and cure for each disease. The extremely successful model works well when doctors care for people with acute infections, such as pneumonia; acute surgical conditions, such as appendicitis; and

Principles of Arthritis Management

1. Each person is an individual with a type of arthritis, but arthritis is not who he or she is.

2. No single "best treatment" exists; individuals respond differently to different treatments.

3. No single type of arthritis is always more or less serious than another type.

4. The information and input a person with arthritis offers can be as valuable for diagnosis and management as information from laboratory tests and X-rays.

5. In arthritis management, the emphasis is on improving the function of joints and relieving pain.

6. Your doctor and health-care team need your involvement to help you. People with arthritis and health professionals are partners in care.

7. Something can always be done to improve life with arthritis.

conditions affecting a single organ, such as a heart attack. Many of our ideas and expectations of medical care stem from this approach, which relies on technologically sophisticated tests and state-of-the-art treatments that lead to cures.

As research on chronic diseases progresses, however, limitations of the biomedical model also become clear. First, the causes and treatments of chronic diseases are complex – there is rarely one cause or one treatment. Second, people who have chronic diseases can contribute to the outcomes of their disease – the results appear to be influenced as much by the actions of the patient as those of the doctor or other health professionals. In fact, growing evidence suggests that much of the key information for making a diagnosis, predicting the outcome and monitoring chronic disease comes from patient histories and questionnaires. These are, of course, supplemented by the knowledge of health professionals and by information gained through medical testing.

As a result, new management strategies have evolved to supplement the traditional biomedical approach. Collectively, the strategies are known as a biopsychosocial model based on the idea that chronic conditions involve many factors – biological, psychological and socioeconomic – that can affect the course and outcome of disease.

The approach emphasizes that people who have chronic diseases should become knowledgeable about the consequences of their disease and the effects of therapy, and they should understand the effect of self-management on disease outcomes. Self-management refers to actions [the patient takes that may favorably affect the course and outcome of chronic disease. By combining self-management strategies with the information and treatment available from doctors and other health professionals, people with arthritis may experience greater benefits – such as increased pain relief and a better quality of life – than those who do not become involved in their own care. Some principles of the biopsychosocial approach are summarized in the box on page 7 and are discussed here. The principles, referred to frequently in the following chapters, create the foundation of this book.

1. Each person is an individual with a type of arthritis, but arthritis is not who he or she is. When a doctor deals with an acute problem, such as a type of pneumonia, the standard course of treatment usually varies little from person to person. Although each patient's case is unique, for acute events, the biomedical model usually works well. However, for a chronic disease such as rheumatoid arthritis, doctors use a more individualized approach. Each person may need a different combination of medications, exercise, therapy and devices to achieve the best quality of life.

2. No single "best treatment" exists; individuals respond differently to different treatments.

In a chronic disease such as arthritis, no single treatment works for all people; each person experiences his or her own symptoms and disease course. In addition, different people may experience different responses to some of the drugs frequently used to treat arthritis. One person may find a medication to be useful, while a second person may get no benefit at all. A third might even have adverse effects from the drug and have to stop taking it. Always ask your health professional about new treatments and whether they might work for you.

3. No single type of arthritis is always more or less serious than another type.

Sometimes people ask, "Is rheumatoid arthritis worse than osteoarthritis?" or the other way around. It's true that, on average, some types of arthritis may cause more pain or disability than other types. However,

arthritis affects each individual differently, and no type of arthritis is invariably better or worse than another type. For example, someone who has bursitis of the hip may experience more discomfort and functional disability than someone with a mild form of rheumatoid arthritis or osteoarthritis.

Some factors that contribute to the severity of the disease include:

- How the condition affects your daily life, including the ability to care for yourself or continue to work;
- How you react to symptoms of pain, fatigue, disability and psychological distress;
- How you respond to treatments, including possible side effects.

Any or all of these can affect how you and the health professionals managing your care perceive the severity of your arthritis.

4. The information and input a person with arthritis offers can be as valuable for diagnosis and management as information from laboratory tests and X-rays.

In the traditional medical approach, doctors rely on tests and data to diagnose and monitor a condition. The tests are often valuable in diagnosing and managing chronic diseases such as rheumatoid arthritis,

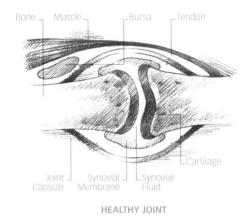

Bone   Muscle   Bursa   Tendon

Joint Capsule   Synovial Membrane   Synovial Fluid   Cartilage

HEALTHY JOINT

but the most important information comes from the patient. In fact, no single test can diagnose or confirm most types of arthritis. You can provide the most important clues through the answers you provide when your doctors takes your patient history. In caring for chronically ill or debilitated people, doctors need to attend to more than just physical symptoms or test results. Your doctor may also use a short questionnaire or diagram to get more information about your arthritis and how it affects your daily life and activities.

5. In arthritis management, the emphasis is on improving the function of joints and relieving pain.

The strategy in many illnesses is to try to get test measures, such as blood pressure, blood sugar (glucose) or cholesterol levels back into a normal range. In rheumatoid arthritis, the strategy is to improve func-

tion, relieve pain, find way to cope and deal with everyday physical and emotional problems related to the disease. Although treatment goals do include getting blood tests, such as an elevated erythrocyte sedimentation rate (ESR or sed rate) or C-reactive protein (CRP) into the normal range (see Chapter 4), your emphasis should be on how you function from day to day – and your daily well-being will likely tell you more about the progress of your treatment than an X-ray or lab test.

6. Your doctor and health-care team need your involvement to help you. People with arthritis and health professionals are partners in care.

If someone is acutely ill, the doctor may be expected to manage the process, such as determining which tests are needed, selecting a treatment and administering these treatments. In a hospital, the doctor writes "orders" and hospital staff provide the treatments. The patient has no responsibility for treatment, other than taking the medicine and cooperating with the prescribed therapy.

When you have a chronic disease, your doctor and other health-care professionals can manage only a small component of your care. You need your doctor to diagnose your illness and prescribe treatment, but since you probably spend less than a few hours each month or even each year with doctors and other health-care professionals, you're in control 99 percent of the time. So, to get the best results, you must be an active participant in your own care. This approach – the cornerstone of this book – is called *self-management*.

The first thing to do if you experience symptoms is to see a doctor and get a proper diagnosis. But once you have that diagnosis, you and your doctor, and other health-care professionals you consult, must act as a team. You – not your doctor – are ultimately in control of whether and when to take a medication, do exercises, practice good joint-protection techniques or take any other steps toward controlling arthritis. Your actions and attitude will determine the success of your treatment.

7. Something can always be done to improve life with arthritis.

You've heard some of the attitudes about life with arthritis: "Arthritis is inevitable," or "Oh, it's arthritis – you can't do anything about it except learn to live with the pain." These attitudes are out of date. Something can always be done to improve a situation for a person with arthritis. It may involve a new drug or surgical technique, a device to make tasks easier, an exercise, a support group or maybe even a book like this one.

Don't expect a miracle. Instead, focus on hard work and determination to make your life with arthritis more productive and enjoyable. Most treatments require some trade-off: time and effort spent on exercise, the cost of a new drug or device, or medication side effects. However, you can be optimistic that your situation can be improved, because it always can.

Chapter 2

Understanding Rheumatoid Arthritis:
A Chronic, Complex Disease

Rheumatoid arthritis (*def.*): A chronic disease in which inflammation of the joints (and sometimes other parts of the body) leads to long-term damage that may result in chronic pain, loss of function and disability.

If you have rheumatoid arthritis, you've probably heard something similar to the definition above from your doctor. Perhaps you have wondered what all these terms mean. In this chapter, we're going to break down this definition into easily understood sections to give you a better understanding of what happens in this complicated condition. We'll also give you some information about the history of rheumatoid arthritis, ongoing research into its possible causes and what it's like to have this disease.

Rheumatoid Arthritis Is Chronic

Rheumatoid arthritis is a chronic disease: once you develop it, it will continue indefinitely. It can begin suddenly or gradually. In some people with rheumatoid arthritis, signs of the arthritis gradually disappear, usually within six months of the onset of symptoms and swelling. This is called spontaneous remission. However, if the pain and swelling continue for longer than six months, you're likely to develop a persistent, or chronic, condition.

Occasionally, people with rheumatoid arthritis may experience bouts of swelling around the joints that occur every few weeks or months, but then subside after a few days. There may be no evidence of any arthritis between these attacks. This is known as *palindromic rheumatism*. (A palindrome is a phrase that reads the same forward and backward, such as "Madam I'm Adam.") About one half of people who experience palindromic rheumatism eventually develop chronic rheumatoid arthritis, including its characteristic persistent inflammation. Others continue to experience limited attacks for many years. In a lucky few, the attacks may even disappear.

Chronic diseases are best diagnosed and monitored through a patient-centered approach: input from the person with arthritis is considered at least as important laboratory tests, perhaps more so. Treatment is complex, usually involving a combination of drugs and other measures over time rather than a single drug. And the person with the illness, using self-help measures, including mind-body approaches, to manage the disease day to day, is a critical part of the disease-management team.

In fact, health-care professionals are generally "in control" of a person's chronic disease less than one-tenth of one percent of the time or less than one hour per month. Most of the time, managing your chronic disease is your responsibility. Learn as much as you can about your disease, its potential course and available treatments. Be proactive in monitoring your symptoms and treatments and in handling the day-to-day challenges your disease brings. Rely on your doctor for treatment prescriptions and advice, but manage your own health and care.

Rheumatoid Arthritis Involves Inflammation

When the body is threatened by some type of foreign invader, such as infection, it normally fights back with inflammation. The body releases chemicals that stimulate fever, swelling and associated pain — signs of inflammation.

In rheumatoid arthritis, inflammation of joints causes them to become swollen, tender and painful. But the inflammation also occurs throughout the body, so organs such as the eyes or lungs may be affected as well. People with rheumatoid arthritis often experience fatigue and flu-like symptoms.

For the most part, the early joint inflammation is reversible. However, if unrecognized and untreated, uncontrolled inflammation — seen as chronic swelling and tenderness of joints — may lead to irreversible joint damage visible on X-rays. Although each person experiences a different disease course, damage may begin in many people as early as the first year of disease. Joint damage caused by inadequately controlled inflammation can lead to loss of joint movement, decreased ability to work, higher medical costs and surgery. That's why getting a diagnosis as soon as possible and beginning a course of drug treatment to control inflammation is so important. Newly developed treatments, such as biologic response modifiers, can control inflammation and prevent joint damage if given early enough in the course of the disease (see Chapter 11).

Rheumatoid Arthritis Involves an Abnormal Immune System Response

Several types of white blood cells are involved in the immune system response. One specialized white blood cell known as a *B-lymphocyte* produces antibodies that neutralize foreign substances known as *antigens*. These antibodies and antigens combine into *immune complexes*, which are then removed by scavenger cells. Another class of cells is called *T-lymphocytes*, which regulate the function of B-cells by suppressing or stimulating the production of antibodies.

The immune system protects the body from disease through an elaborate network of signals that control the production of antibodies. Normally, this system works very well to maintain your health. But in rheumatoid arthritis, the signals don't function properly. The immune system mistakenly views the body as the foreign invader, a process known as *autoimmunity*. The immune cells then attack the body, causing inflammation that later results in damage to joints and other organs.

One example of the erring signals involves a type of "anti-antibody" known as *rheumatoid factor* that regulates other normal antibodies. Rheumatoid factor in small quantities may act normally. However, people with excess amounts of rheumatoid factor may have immune systems that do not function properly.

Although most people with rheumatoid arthritis do have rheumatoid factor, it may not be detected early in the disease. And some people with severe rheumatoid arthritis never have rheumatoid factor. However, the discovery of rheumatoid factor has led to recent advances in treatments, establishing that the immune system in those with rheumatoid arthritis is incorrectly programmed.

The immune system has been — and continues to be — the subject of much research. Many potential therapies for rheumatoid arthritis and other autoimmune diseases aim to correct the faulty signals that distort the immune response and to overcome their consequences.

Who Gets Rheumatoid Arthritis?

Rheumatoid arthritis affects about 0.5 percent

to 1 percent of the population in the United States and most countries around the world. That's about 2.1 million Americans. Rheumatoid arthritis may begin at any age. It affects infants, the elderly, and those in their prime. However, more than 70 percent of people with rheumatoid arthritis are women, and the most common onset is between the ages of 40 and 50.

What Causes Rheumatoid Arthritis?

Despite extensive research, the cause of rheumatoid arthritis remains unknown. Scientists have learned much about the immune response and the mechanisms of inflammation in arthritis (see the beginning of this chapter), but the events that start the abnormal process remain a mystery.

Historically, doctors have considered RA a chronic infectious arthritis because its features are similar to those of infectious diseases like tuberculosis. However, scientists have failed to identify a specific infectious agent (such as a bacterium, fungus or virus). More recently, researchers have tried to identify the footprints of an agent (such as the genetic material or DNA of an infectious agent) in the tissue of people with rheumatoid arthritis. To date, these studies remain inconclusive.

Even if the footprints of such an agent –

or the agent itself – were consistently found in people with rheumatoid arthritis, it is unlikely that everyone infected with the agent would get rheumatoid arthritis. Genetic makeup influences whether or not an individual develops an infection from any agent, even the common flu virus. So even if most people with rheumatoid arthritis carry an infectious agent, that explains only part of the reason why they develop the disease. Other factors contribute.

What is now called rheumatoid arthritis may actually include many different diseases. Such surprises have happened many times in the history of medicine. For instance, 150 years ago physicians recognized only a few types of pneumonia. Today, they recognize dozens.

The Role of Gender

One important clue about the origin of rheumatoid arthritis is gender. As noted earlier, more than 70 percent of people with rheumatoid arthritis are women. This observation has led to theories that gender may play some part in what causes rheumatoid arthritis and its severity.

Many women with rheumatoid arthritis experience improvement in their symptoms during pregnancy. And after a baby is born, women may experience an

Personally Speaking STORIES FROM REAL PEOPLE

"I was diagnosed in October 2003 with rheumatoid arthritis. I suffered for three years beginning the day after the birth of my son. After years of inaccurate diagnoses and limping around in horrible pain for more than six months, I was finally diagnosed with rheumatoid arthritis.

"I've tried several treatments, and I'm currently on *Remicade*. I am a 36-year-old female who has always been active and in good health. To help ease my pain, I take yoga classes and exercise regularly using my treadmill and other light floor exercises.

AFTER DIAGNOSIS: I KEEP MOVING
— CARLENE FIORITO, EAST PROVIDENCE, RI

"My husband and family have been very support-ive. They often help me with housework and keep my spirits up with their concern and care. If it weren't for my twin sister who helps me in every way, I'm not sure where I would be. I also read a lot and I'm active in my treatment. I constantly do research, look-ing for helpful tips about how to live and cope with RA. I eat a healthy diet, drink no caffeine, and even when I feel like I can't get out of bed because of severe fatigue, I keep moving!

"My faith in God and something much bigger than me gets me through each and every day."

increase in symptoms. Furthermore, rheumatoid arthritis develops more often than expected in the year after a pregnancy. However, the understanding of the effects of female hormones in rheumatoid arthri-tis remains limited.

The Role of Other Genetic Factors

Over the last 20 years, progress has been made toward identifying genes linked to an increased risk of developing rheuma-toid arthritis. One such factor found on the surface of lymphocytes, or white blood cells, is known as *major histocom-patibility antigen*, or *human lymphocyte antigen* (HLA). The HLA genetic site, or locus, controls immune responses. Researchers have shown that people with a specific genetic marker called *HLA shared epitope* have a fivefold greater probability of developing rheumatoid arthritis than people without the marker. More than two-thirds of Caucasian people with rheumatoid arthritis have this genetic marker, compared to only about 20 percent of the general population.

Although this genetic marker is associated with increased risk of disease and may be an important clue in the cause of rheumatoid arthritis, it cannot be used as a diagnostic test: only a small minority of people with the shared epitope develop rheumatoid arthritis. In addition, many people with rheumatoid arthritis do not have this genetic marker.

Further research suggests that other, yet-to-be-identified genes influence the development of disease as well. Researchers continue to search for these genes by identifying families in which several members have arthritis and analyzing their DNA (which makes up the genetic code).

New Insights

New research suggests that stress may play a role in rheumatoid arthritis. Stress can refer to a physical trauma, emotional upheaval or anything that stimulates the body to produce a stress response. Some researchers have suggested that rheumatoid arthritis may begin or worsen at times of stress.

Normally, the central nervous system responds to stress by sending out a compli-

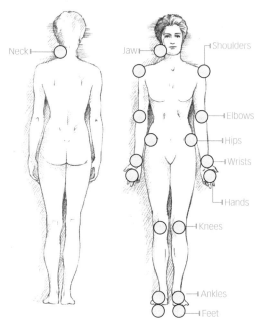

JOINTS THAT MAY BE AFFECTED
BY RHEUMATOID ARTHRITIS

cated series of signals resulting in the production of corticosteroids, or anti-inflammatory hormones, by the body's adrenal glands. So a stressful stimulus should lead to an increase in corticosteroid levels. However, some people with rheumatoid arthritis appear to have a blunted response to stress, causing them to produce lower levels of corticosteroids. This may explain why people with rheumatoid arthritis often respond well to small doses of corticosteroid drugs such as prednisone.

What is it Like to Have Rheumatoid Arthritis?

All this information about the process of

inflammation and what happens inside your body at a cellular level doesn't tell you what RA feels like on a daily basis. So, what follows is a description of the symptoms you *may* experience with the disease; the problems of one person may differ greatly from those of another. The most common symptoms of RA include:

- Stiffness (especially in the morning)
- Fatigue
- Pain
- Swelling in multiple joints

While any joint may become involved, many people first experience symptoms of joint inflammation in the knuckles of the hands, feet and wrists. In some people with RA, the elbows, shoulders, hips and knees become involved as well.

A summary of the joints most likely affected can be found in the diagram on the opposite page. In addition, the box below provides definitions that will help you understand the structure of your joints and how they are affected by inflammation.

In addition to physical symptoms, people with RA often experience psychological stress, frustration, helplessness and loss of

Your Joints: A Marvel of Engineering

A joint connects one bone to another. Joints come in various shapes and sizes: some move like a hinge (your finger and knee joints, for example); others have a "ball in socket" structure that allows them to move in many directions (your shoulder and hip joints); still others only move in several directions (your wrist and ankle). There are more than 70 moveable joints in the body – and rheumatoid arthritis can affect any of them.

Other soft-tissue structures surround the joint and may also be affected by arthritis. Ligaments are flexible bands of fibrous tissue that connect bones to one another. Muscles consist of fibers that stretch and tighten, allowing movement of the body's organs and joints. At the ends of muscles are tendons that connect muscle to bone.

If you looked inside a joint, you would find cartilage, a smooth substance that lines the joint so your bones do not wear each other down. The synovial fluid produced by the synovium, or lining of the joint, lubricates it and allows free movement. When joints are inflamed, inflammatory cells are found in the synovial fluid and lining, and cause breakdown of cartilage and bone.

control as they learn to cope with the day-to-day effects of this chronic disease. Psychological problems can, in turn, make coping with arthritis more difficult and even increase pain. The good news is that you can do something about the cycle of pain and depression. Getting proper treatments and developing new skills – on your own or with the help of others – to cope with pain and stress in positive, constructive ways can help you fight that spiraling cycle.

Although arthritis is a chronic disease, you can control your symptoms. And the severe consequences of rheumatoid arthritis may now be prevented in most people.

Drugs now are more effective and have fewer side effects than traditional medications. Used early in the disease and in combination with one another, these can bring about more effective control of inflammation. Exercise programs, joint protection activities and self-management techniques can also help people take control. All of these strategies will be discussed later in this book.

So, stay informed, be active about your care, but above all, be optimistic. People with rheumatoid arthritis can feel more optimistic about their future than ever before. You can achieve good living with rheumatoid arthritis.

Chapter 3

Diagnosing Rheumatoid Arthritis:
Your Medical History and Physical Examination

Diagnosis is the first step on the road to proper treatment and control of rheumatoid arthritis. RA symptoms often occur suddenly, causing confusion for the person affected. As no single laboratory test can instantly confirm an RA diagnosis, doctors must use a variety of methods to determine the cause of patients' symptoms. The more you know about these methods and the importance of the information you provide, the better you will be at understanding and participating in the process.

RA differs from other diseases such as diabetes or kidney disease, which can be diagnosed in most people by simple blood tests. By contrast, the rheumatoid factor – the antibody that may indicate rheumatoid arthritis – (see the previous chapter) test is positive in many people with rheumatoid arthritis, but negative in 20 to 30 percent of the people who have this disease. And a test for rheumatoid factor may be positive in people who do not have rheumatoid arthritis.

Even discovering which type of arthritis a person has is not always easy. As we discussed in Chapter 1, each person experiences his or her own disease course, and a person may have more than one type of rheumatic condition at the same time. A skilled physician will use the information provided by the patient and the findings of a physical examination to make a preliminary diagnosis and then determine which tests are needed. In fact, the most important parts of the diagnostic process are a careful medical history, including a full discussion of current symptoms, and a complete physical exam. Tests do not always provide a clear answer.

The "Low-Tech" Tools

Medicine now routinely incorporates highly advanced technology and devices in its practice. Batteries of tests and the use of expensive imaging equipment have become standard. However, the most important and perhaps surprising tools for the diagnosis of rheumatoid arthritis are the less technical components of your office visit – your medical history and physical examination.

Medical History

Ever wonder why you have to fill out forms and answer so many questions when you visit your doctor? No, it's not just a plot to distract you while you wait for the nurse to call you in – you're actually providing important clues that help your doctor make a diagnosis. Some of the key questions he or she may ask during your initial office visit include:

• **Do you have joint pain in many joints?** People who have rheumatoid arthritis usually experience joint involvement in several joints at once, as opposed to having pain in only one joint.

• **Does the pain occur symmetrically – that is, do the same joints on both sides of your body hurt at the same time?** Or is the pain one-sided? Symmetric pain is often a sign of rheumatoid arthritis. For

instance, if both wrists or the same knuckles in both hands are swollen, rheumatoid arthritis may be likely.

• **Do you have stiffness in the morning?** Morning stiffness, another hallmark of rheumatoid arthritis, occurs when the joints feel stiff and are difficult to move. Doctors are often interested in how long your morning stiffness lasts. After a period of loosening up, motion becomes easier and less painful. Stiffness is likely to recur after sitting for prolonged periods of time.

• **When is the pain most severe?** For example, do your joints hurt more in the morning or late in the day? When you have rheumatoid arthritis, your joints often feel better with moderate activity, but you may be most uncomfortable in early morning and again later in the day as fatigue sets in.

• **Do you have pain in your hands, wrists and/or feet?** Although rheumatoid arthritis can occur in any joint of the body, these joints are most frequently involved, growing painful and swollen.

• **If you do have pain in your hands, which joints hurt the most?** In rheumatoid arthritis, rows of joints – for example, the knuckles that join your fingers to your hand (metacarpophalangeal joints) and the middle knuckles of the fingers (proximal interphalangeal joints) – tend to be affected more often than the knuckles near the tips of the fingers.

- **Have you had periods of feeling weak and uncomfortable all over?** Do you feel fatigued? Many people with rheumatoid arthritis notice generalized problems, such as muscle aches, fatigue, stiffness, weight loss and a general "flu-like" feeling.

Your answers to these and other questions often let the doctor know if rheumatoid arthritis should be considered as a diagnosis. And, if you have already been diagnosed with rheumatoid arthritis, your medical history will continue to play a starring role in your office visits since your doctor will want to keep tabs on your pain and functional status, any developing limitations in your movements and activities, your medications, and any side effects.

Patient Questionnaires

Doctors increasingly use self-report questionnaires, in addition to medical history, to glean critical information about the course of your disease and treatment. Some of the most important problems experienced by people with rheumatoid arthritis, including loss of function, pain, fatigue and psychological distress, cannot be measured by any blood test, X-ray or other high-tech measure. So, doctors use the results from patient questionnaires to assess the impact of rheumatoid arthritis on daily life.

If your doctor is not currently using a patient questionnaire, you may want to discuss that with him or her since these measures are one of the most effective ways to monitor changes in disease over a five- to 10-year period. Two of the most common self-report questionnaires used in the care of those with rheumatoid arthritis are described below.

- **The Health Assessment Questionnaire (HAQ).** This measurement tool includes 20 activities of daily living in eight categories including dressing, eating, walking and other activities. Participants are also asked to measure their pain and overall outlook, and to answer questions about their use of aids and devices. Two-page modified versions (modified HAQ, and multidimensional HAQ) have been developed to provide additional data that includes global status, measures of fatigue and psychological distress, and medication review.

- **The Arthritis Impact Measurement Scales (AIMS).** This tool measures several dimensions of health status including mobility, physical activity, dexterity, household activities, anxiety, depression and social activities, in addition to activities of daily living and pain.

28

"I had only been married about six months when my symptoms – extreme pain in my wrists and ankles – started. I was fatigued all of the time. I had no energy. I'm a first grade teacher, and my job requires constant attention to my students. I had to stay on my feet and I barely had enough energy to make it through the day.

"I went to several doctors trying to find out what my problem was. My doctor said I was depressed. But I knew my body better than anyone else, and I knew my problems were more than depression. Yes, I was depressed because no one could tell me what my physical problem was.

STARTING OVER: A FIRST
GRADE TEACHER'S TALE
– SHERRY COLLIER,
WYLLIESBURG, VA

"After many tests, my doctor referred me to a rheumatologist who did more tests and finally concluded that I had RA. He started me on medicine that has helped me work every day. Sometimes the days are long but I do my best to hang in there.

"Not only do I have RA, but I have also been diagnosed with multiple sclerosis. Each day is a challenge. But I am fortunate: I have a wonderful family that has been there for me throughout this long ordeal. I give thanks also to my doctor who never gave up on finding the cause of my problems. Most of all, I thank God for each new day and the strength to see me through."

Physical Examination

After taking your medical history, a doctor knowledgeable about rheumatoid arthritis should give you a thorough physical examination that supplies most of the necessary information to make a diagnosis. Your doctor will look for common features of RA, including:

• **Joint swelling.** This may be severe or barely noticeable. A skilled doctor should be able to recognize even slight joint swelling that may indicate rheumatoid arthritis.

• **Joint tenderness.** Certain joints may be painful to even the slightest touch.

• **Loss of motion in your joints.** This may indicate inflammation (see Chapter 2 for a description of the inflammatory process) or joint damage. The physician will assess your joints' range of motion, asking questions such as, "Can you move your shoulders through a complete circle?"

- **Joint malalignment.** After several years of rheumatoid arthritis (especially if inflammation is unchecked), some joint damage often occur s– most commonly in the small joints of the hands and feet – causing joints to be out of alignment.
- **Signs of rheumatoid arthritis in other organs.** Rheumatoid arthritis is a systemic disease, meaning it may affect multiple systems in your body. The doctor will look for involvement in your skin, lungs and eyes, and other parts of your body.

The doctor will review each joint during the physical exam to determine which joints have signs of arthritis, including tenderness, pain during motion, swelling, limited motion and long-term damage. Knowing the number of affected joints is useful in assessing, monitoring and predicting the course of rheumatoid arthritis. Usually, your doctor will not only count the involved joints but will also assess the severity of RA in each joint.

Physical Measures of Function

Your doctor may want to get an idea of your ability to perform certain tasks. Measures of your physical function may indicate both evidence of inflammation and evidence of long-term damage. A member of your doctor's office staff, or a physical or occupational therapist may perform these tests. Some widely used measures include:

- **Grip strength.** The traditional method for measuring grip strength has been to inflate a blood pressure cuff (30 mmHg) and ask the individual to squeeze as hard as possible, first with the right then with the left hand. The pressure change on the cuff is recorded. The test is usually repeated several times.
- **Walking time.** The individual is asked to walk a set distance (usually 25 or 50 feet) at a normal pace. The time to complete the distance is then recorded.
- **Button test.** The individual is asked to unbutton and button five buttons as quickly as possible using a standard button board. The score is recorded in seconds.

Classification Criteria

You may have heard or read about something called *classification criteria for rheumatoid arthritis.* (See box, next page.) They were developed by a committee of rheumatologists (doctors who specialize in treating arthritis) and provide a guideline of the patterns usually seen in rheumatoid arthritis.

Summary

As you can see, your doctor is able to obtain most of the valuable information needed to make a diagnosis of rheumatoid arthritis before a laboratory test is ever ordered. Your contribution can be substantial when you provide clear and accurate information about your medical history, as well as any family history of arthritis or joint symptoms. Keep track of which joints have been swollen or painful, because the disease may over time abate in some joints and flare in others.

Lab tests can provide important additional information for a diagnosis. We'll discuss these tests in the next chapter.

Classification Criteria for Rheumatoid Arthritis

These classification criteria were developed by members of the American College of Rheumatology. They describe patterns of symptoms that are most commonly seen in people with rheumatoid arthritis. They can be used as guidelines, but they will not give you or your doctor specific information about your prognosis (what will happen over time with your condition).

Classification Criteria

1. Morning stiffness

2. Arthritis of three or more joints

3. Arthritis of more than two hand joints

4. Symmetrical arthritis

5. Subcutaneous (rheumatoid) nodules

6. Rheumatoid factor

7. Radiographic (X-ray) changes

Adapted from "Revised Classification Criteria for Rheumatoid Arthritis," *Arthritis and Rheumatism*, 1988, Volume 31, pp. 315-324, by Arnett, Edworthy, Bloch, et al.

Chapter 4

Diagnosing Rheumatoid Arthritis:
Laboratory Tests and Imaging Studies

Like puzzle pieces, the information and clues that you and your doctor uncover will fit together, helping to determine whether or not you have rheumatoid arthritis. As you know from previous chapters, no laboratory test can absolutely determine whether or not you have rheumatoid arthritis.

People with rheumatoid arthritis can have normal test results, and people can have abnormal test results yet not have rheumatoid arthritis. Interpretation of laboratory tests depends on the symptoms of the individual. So answering your doctor's questions honestly is essential.

Some of the tests discussed in this chapter may be familiar to you. Others are used less commonly and may not be necessary for you. At times you may feel that you are looking into a bowl of alphabet soup as you ponder the importance of your ESR, RF, ANA and MRI, among others. But all of these tests can provide important clues when used in the right way.

When Tests Are Helpful

Laboratory tests and imaging procedures can help your doctor confirm your diagnosis. In addition, they may help determine the severity of disease activity. Your doctor may choose to order only one or two tests discussed in the chapter, or he or she may use a test not described here. In general, you will not repeat most tests after a diagnosis is made. Other tests, designed to check for drug side effects or to measure improvement, may need to be repeated regularly.

Laboratory Tests Used in Diagnosis
Complete Blood Count

Doctors measure levels, or counts, of different types of blood cells to assess patients with many types of diseases. Blood is composed of three cellular components: red blood cells carry oxygen to tissues, white blood cells help the body fight infections, and platelets help stop bleeding and form clots. Doctors often measure these cells during your first office visit. They may repeat this test during treatment to check for drug side effects and to monitor any progress in reversing abnormalities.

Doctors evaluate red blood cells by looking at measures of hemoglobin, and the number and volume of red blood cells. Hemoglobin is the protein in red blood cells that carries oxygen from the lungs to the tissues. It may be low in those with rheumatoid arthritis, a result of the anemia, or lower than normal number of red blood cells, common in RA. The ratio of the volume of red blood cells to the volume of whole blood is called the *hematocrit*. Both the volume, or hematocrit, and the number of red blood cells, or red blood cell count, may be lower than normal in people with rheumatoid arthritis. That anemia in some people with rheumatoid arthritis may contribute to feelings of fatigue or malaise. People with a more aggressive level of the disease tend to have more severe anemia.

Your doctor may also periodically count the level of your white blood cells. A high white cell count may mean that an infection is present and can be a sign of severe inflammation. However, the white blood cell count is usually normal in people with rheumatoid arthritis, unless a simultaneous infection is present. (The white cell count may also be low from an unusual complication of rheumatoid arthritis called *Felty's syndrome*, which we'll discuss later.) Some of the medications used to treat rheumatoid arthritis may cause a reduction in the white cell count, thereby reducing the body's capacity to fight infections.

Platelets are small cells involved in the formation of blood clots. Severe inflammation may elevate the platelet count, and certain drugs may depress it. The platelet count, along with the white blood cell count, are monitored about every six months in people who take nonsteroidal anti-inflammatory drugs (NSAIDs), such as ibuprofen and naproxen, and about every two to 12 weeks in people who take most disease-modifying antirheumatic drugs (DMARDs), such as methotrexate and leflunomide.

Erythrocyte Sedimentation Rate

The erythrocyte sedimentation rate, also known as *ESR* or *sed rate*, is a measure of inflammation. The hour-long test calculates how fast red blood cells (erythrocytes) fall to the bottom of a glass tube filled with blood. People with any type of inflammation, including rheumatoid arthritis, often have higher sed rates than those without inflammation. If treatment reduces the inflammation, the sed rate usually drops. Because it is so important to control inflammation in rheumatoid arthritis, doctors may repeat this test fairly frequently.

One problem is that the ESR is elevated in only about 60 percent of people who have rheumatoid arthritis, meaning that the remaining 40 percent have a normal sedimentation rate. Your treatment is generally directed by the severity of your clinical symptoms, such as pain and functional ability. So, even if your ESR is normal, treatment for your rheumatoid arthritis often should continue.

C-Reactive Protein

C-reactive protein (or CRP) is another substance found in the body that indicates the presence of inflammation. Elevated levels of this protein provide an additional measure of disease activity in rheumatoid arthritis. Although the ESR and CRP often reflect similar degrees of inflammation, sometimes ESR levels are elevated when CRP levels are normal (and vice versa). This phenomenon is not well understood.

Some researchers have recognized that CRP levels that remain high over a long period are often associated with more severe joint damage later in the disease. This provides a strong rationale for trying to reduce CRP levels to normal. However, some people with normal levels may still experience progressive joint damage.

As with the sedimentation rate, treatment for rheumatoid arthritis usually should continue even if CRP levels are normal. Your doctor may repeat this test regularly to monitor the level of inflammation and your response to medication.

Rheumatoid Factor

Rheumatoid factor (RF) is an antibody found in the blood of about 70 percent to 80 percent of people with rheumatoid arthritis. These abnormal antibodies are proteins produced by B-lymphocytes, or particular white blood cells, in response to substances such as infectious agents. And they are often found in the blood serum of people with rheumatoid arthritis. Blood serum, blood's liquid component, makes up about half of the blood; red blood cells, white blood cells and platelets make up the other half. As discussed in Chapter 2, rheumatoid factor in small quantities regulates normal antibodies produced by the body, known as gamma globulins or immunoglobulin G (IgG).

Most people with rheumatoid arthritis have a large amount of rheumatoid factor circulating in the blood. However, the rheumatoid factor test is not a specific diagnostic test for rheumatoid arthritis. At least one in five people with rheumatoid arthritis does not have rheumatoid factor, but does have a form of the disease that cannot be distinguished from the disease in those who do have rheumatoid factor.

People with rheumatoid arthritis who do not have rheumatoid factor in their serum are often referred to as *seronegative*. As noted, their disease doesn't differ from that of *seropositive* people, or those who do have rheumatoid factor. The rheumatoid factor test, also called the *rheumatoid arthritis latex test*, measures the amount of these antibodies in titers or units. A titer is a number indicating the dilution of blood at which rheumatoid factor may be detected; if a titer is 1:160, the serum contains twice as much rheumatoid factor than a titer of 1:80. Rheumatoid factor may also be measured in units, and higher numbers mean more rheumatoid factor. However, test results may be negative during the first sev-

eral months that you have the disease, making the test less useful in early diagnosis. Nonetheless, the test for rheumatoid factor is eventually positive in 60 percent to 80 percent of people with rheumatoid arthritis.

Experts once thought that people with RA who had a positive rheumatoid factor test were more likely to have a severe disease course. Recent studies suggest that the differences in disease severity between those who do and do not have rheumatoid factor are not necessarily as great as researchers once believed.

Antinuclear Antibodies

Another test for abnormal antibodies is called the *antinuclear antibody (ANA) test*. It detects autoantibodies (proteins that attack certain tissues or organs) that combine with the nuclei of cells. These antibodies are most often positive in people with systemic lupus erythematosus (also known as SLE or lupus), but they also appear in about 30 to 40 percent of people with rheumatoid arthritis. A positive ANA test may be seen in people with scleroderma (systemic sclerosis), polymyositis and other inflammatory rheumatic diseases as well.

Most people with positive antinuclear antibody tests have neither rheumatoid arthritis nor lupus, however, and probably

"When I felt foot pain followed by wrist pain, I suspected I might have RA. I was no stranger to the condition. My mother has it, as did my grandfather and great-grand-father. So, I had some inside information.

"I started treatments soon after my diagnosis by a rheumatologist. Still, my activities and abilities were affected. I had to teach my high-school history classes in bed-room slippers and ask students to carry my book bag from my car to my classroom. I was able to continue teaching full time for four more years. But aerobics and skiing were replaced by walking my dog and swimming.

AGGRESSIVE APPROACH: SIMPLE COPING, STRONG SUPPORT
– LINDA SHULL, CHARLOTTE, NC

"My strategies for coping are simple. RA is the hand I have been dealt. My family and friends have been essential for my success in living well with RA. When I told my husband (one month after our wedding) that I would need a hip replacement, he became the solid rock of support I knew he would be. His steadfastness in 'sickness and health' was tested far earlier than he expected, but his love and compassion have never wavered.

"Also, close friends circled the wagons and tirelessly volunteered comfort, cheer and understanding. They signed up for the harder labor – cooking, cleaning and taxi service – whenever I needed them. Overall, I have chosen to live as normally as my health permits. I have made RA a part of my life, not the focus of my life. I am blessed that I have many people in my life who help me do that every day."

have no disease at all. Because of the difficulty of interpreting results, many doctors no longer routinely use this test.

Genetic Typing

In recent years, attention has been focused on the search for genetic markers that may predispose certain people to develop or be susceptible to a particular disease. About two-thirds of people with rheumatoid arthritis have a genetic marker known as a *shared epitope* (see Chapter 2) located where the genes that control the immune system response are.

Although identification of this shared epitope is critical for research studies to understand how rheumatoid arthritis develops, about seven percent of the well population have the marker but do not develop rheumatoid arthritis. And at least 20 percent of people with rheumatoid arthritis do not have the shared epitope. So measurement of the epitope is not useful in diagnosing rheumatoid arthritis.

Urinalysis

A routine study of urine (urinalysis or UA) includes tests for sugar (which can identify and monitor diabetes), protein (seen when kidney abnormalities are present), and abnormal cells that indicate inflammation or infection of the kidney, bladder or other parts of the urinary tract. A urinalysis is not helpful in the diagnosis of rheumatoid arthritis, but it is used regularly in people with rheumatoid arthritis who are treated with certain medications such as gold or penicillamine. These drugs may cause damage to the kidneys, so monitoring is necessary.

Imaging Studies
Radiographs (X-rays)

X-rays taken early in the course of rheumatoid arthritis can show swelling of soft tissues and loss of bone density around the joints stemming from reduced activity and inflammation. In later stages, about 70 percent of people with rheumatoid arthritis develop erosions (small holes) near the ends of their bones and a narrowing of joint space due to cartilage loss.

Doctors once believed that they should delay aggressive drug treatment of RA until erosions – which confirm a rheumatoid arthritis diagnosis – were visible because of the potential side effects of the drugs. Today, doctors use the opposite approach, treating RA early and aggressively before damage appears. So X-rays are not necessarily used as guides to initiate treatment, but they remain important in evaluating how well treatments control joint damage and when people may need joint surgery.

X-rays taken early in the disease course can also provide a valuable baseline for comparison with later X-rays to see if and how the disease has progressed. People with rheumatoid arthritis should have X-rays of the hands and feet every one to two years.

Bone Scans

Bone scans may be used to detect evidence of inflammation in the body, including joints. Although bone scans may be used to confirm the presence of polyarthritis (arthritis affecting multiple joints), this condition can usually be detected in a physical examination. So, bone scans are generally not necessary to make a diagnosis of rheumatoid arthritis.

Magnetic Resonance Imaging (MRI)

MRI scanning is becoming an important diagnostic aid and monitor of arthritis activity in the joints. And it can detect early inflammation before it appears on an X-ray. The scans are also effective at pinpointing synovitis (inflammation of the lining of the joint) in many people who show no damage on X-rays.

Joint Ultrasound

Joint ultrasound is a much less expensive way than MRIs to look for joint inflam-

mation before X-rays show damage. Although not currently used often, doctors may use the procedure more often over the next few years as they increase efforts to document early evidence of disease.

Bone Densitometry

Some doctors suggest that a bone density test, or bone densitometry, should be part of the evaluation and monitoring of all people with rheumatoid arthritis, particularly for women after menopause. Doctors use the imaging study primarily to detect osteoporosis – a major clinical problem for older people, particularly women. Osteoporosis may be especially severe in people with rheumatoid arthritis due to joint immobilization, the inflammatory response itself, and the use of certain therapies (corticosteroids) that may hasten bone loss.

Chapter 5

Diagnosis Checkpoints:
What if it's not Rheumatoid Arthritis?

For the majority of people with rheumatoid arthritis, establishing a diagnosis can be done with confidence. But even skilled rheumatologists on occasion may have difficulty determining whether a person has rheumatoid arthritis or one of several other diseases that can have similar symptoms.

Diagnosis is not always a simple journey to a clear destination. When large groups of patients are studied over long periods, about five percent of people originally diagnosed with rheumatoid arthritis discover five to 10 years later that they have another type of rheumatic disease. Another five percent of people diagnosed with other rheumatic diseases may turn out to have rheumatoid arthritis.

What is recognized today as rheumatoid arthritis probably involves many different types of diseases (see Chapter 1). In the future, physicians may well be able to distinguish several different forms of rheumatoid arthritis. This may partly explain why a diagnosis of rheumatoid arthritis can vary in the number of affected joints or organs, the severity of symptoms, and the way the disease responds to therapy.

In this chapter, we take a look at some of the many other types of rheumatic diseases whose symptoms can sometimes mimic or resemble rheumatoid arthritis (see "Diseases That Can Resemble Rheumatoid Arthritis," page 44). Some of these diseases can even occur with rheumatoid arthritis, making it even more important to obtain an accurate diagnosis and appropriate treatment.

Osteoarthritis

Osteoarthritis (sometimes called degenerative joint disease) occurs when joint

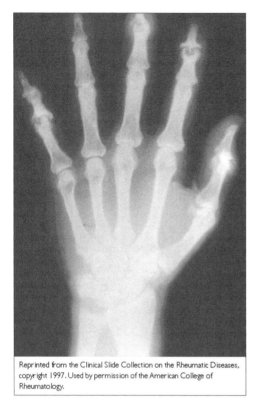

Reprinted from the Clinical Slide Collection on the Rheumatic Diseases, copyright 1997. Used by permission of the American College of Rheumatology.

EROSIVE OSTEOARTHRITIS

cartilage is worn away, causing damage and eventual destruction of the joint. This condition was once thought to be an inevitable part of getting old, and certainly the chance of developing it increases with age. However, many people never develop osteoarthritis, and many people with osteoarthritis do not show any additional progression for five to 10 years. New research suggests that active mechanisms – not just aging and its accompanying processes – play a part in the development of osteoarthritis.

It is usually a simple matter to distinguish between osteoarthritis and rheumatoid arthritis. Some forms of osteoarthritis, however, can look like rheumatoid arthritis. Erosive osteoarthritis, for example, results in bony enlargement of the middle hand knuckle joints and/or the knuckles closest to the tips of the fingers. On X-rays, erosions can look very much like those in rheumatoid arthritis. The knuckles nearest the wrist are generally not involved in erosive osteoarthritis, however, which provides one way to distinguish this form of osteoarthritis from rheumatoid arthritis (see the image, this page). Furthermore, unlike rheumatoid arthritis, the wrists, elbows and ankles generally are not involved in erosive osteoarthritis.

Occasionally, people develop osteoarthritis that is symmetric (affects the same joints on both sides of the body), a hallmark of rheumatoid arthritis. This may be seen primarily in both hands, hips or knees.

Sometimes when a joint already has extensive damage from the inflammatory process of rheumatoid arthritis, but the inflammation itself is no longer present, the doctor may not be sure whether the damage was caused by osteoarthritis or rheumatoid arthritis. However, a detailed patient history and examination of other joints will usually allow the physician to determine the cause. Still, at this point, the cause is less important than addressing the damage itself (for instance, through joint replacement surgery).

Fibromyalgia

Fibromyalgia is a syndrome that, like rheumatoid arthritis, is more common among women – about 90 percent of people with fibromyalgia are women, compared with 70 percent of people with rheumatoid arthritis. The most common symptom is widespread, generalized musculoskeletal pain, which may occur in the back, shoulders, neck or any other part of the body. This widespread pain may raise a concern that the patient has rheumatoid arthritis, but fibromyalgia causes no swelling or other evidence of inflammation in the joints.

People with fibromyalgia often have a history of sleep difficulties, and they may also experience problems in other organ systems, such as migraine headaches or irritable bowel syndrome. These are not

Disease Differences

Osteoarthritis	Rheumatoid Arthritis
Usually begins after age 40	Usually begins between ages 15 and 50
Usually develops over many years	May develop within weeks or months
Affects a few joints and may occur on both sides of the body	Usually affects many joints, primarily the small joints on both sides of the body
Joint redness, warmth and swelling is usually minimal. Morning stiffness is common and may be severe but brief	Causes redness, warmth, swelling and prolonged morning stiffness of the joints
Affects only certain joints, most commonly hips, knees and lower back	Affects many joints, most commonly hands, wrists and feet
Doesn't cause a general feeling of sickness and fatigue	Often causes a general feeling of sickness and fatigue, as well as weight loss and fever

associated with damage to the body, but can cause severe distress.

Although people with fibromyalgia may experience joint tenderness, the tenderness usually encompasses muscle groups (for example, muscles of the head and neck; muscles of the legs, etc.). However, people with rheumatoid arthritis may not have joint swelling at times, and they may show evidence of fibromyalgia. It appears that fibromyalgia is considerably more common in people with rheumatoid arthritis than in the general population – and in fact, some people have both rheumatoid arthritis and fibromyalgia. When this happens, both conditions may be mild, or one may be mild and the other severe.

Distinguishing whether rheumatoid arthritis or fibromyalgia may account for symptoms is important because drugs used to treat rheumatoid arthritis usually do not help the symptoms of fibromyalgia. However, because many symptoms are common in both rheumatoid arthritis and fibromyalgia, including generalized muscle pain, morning stiffness, difficulty sleeping soundly and fatigue, the doctor and patient must sometimes make an educated guess about the likely cause of particular symptoms.

Diseases That Can Resemble Rheumatoid Arthritis

| Osteoarthritis * |
| Fibromyalgia* |
| Gout |
| Ankylosing spondylitis |
| Bursitis and Tendinitis* |
| Sjögren's syndrome* |
| Felty's syndrome * |
| Polymyalgia rheumatica |
| Connective Tissue Diseases: |
| Systemic lupus erythematosus (lupus) |
| Scleroderma |
| Polymyositis/Dermatomyositis |
| Vasculitis |

*indicates disease/syndromes that occur commonly with rheumatoid arthritis.

Gout

Gout has been called "the great masquerader" because it can mimic almost any other rheumatic disease. Gout occurs when an excess of uric acid leads to the formation of crystals in the joint. The crystals can form deposits called *tophi* in the joints. These can stimulate an inflammatory response that can cause an extremely painful attack of arthritis. Although gout (once called *podagra*) most often occurs in the big toe, it can involve virtually any joint or joints and, in time, the attacks may become chronic and resemble rheumatoid arthritis.

Certain features help distinguish gout from rheumatoid arthritis. First, gout usually occurs in men, whereas rheumatoid arthritis is more common in women. Second, gout usually does not involve the hands (at least in early stages of the disease), but rheumatoid arthritis does. Third, most of the pain and inflammation from gout occurs in episodes, rather than continually as in rheumatoid arthritis.

Distinguishing between gout and rheumatoid arthritis is important because medications that can lower uric acid levels and control gout attacks differ from those used to treat rheumatoid arthritis.

Ankylosing Spondylitis

Ankylosing spondylitis is another generalized form of arthritis that can resemble rheumatoid arthritis. Joints commonly involved are those of the back, neck, shoulders, hips and knees. Rheumatoid arthritis tends to affect the small joints of the hands and feet. As with gout, ankylosing spondylitis is more common among men; rheumatoid arthritis is seen more often in women.

Although ankylosing spondylitis is a systemic disease like rheumatoid arthritis, it does not usually cause as much fatigue or lack of well-being. The inflammation in ankylosing spondylitis occurs in the enthesis – the place where the tendon inserts itself into the bone – as well as in the lining of the joint, just as in rheumatoid arthritis. People with ankylosing spondylitis tend to respond to different drugs and exercise programs than those with RA, and these treatment differences reinforce the importance of a correct diagnosis.

Researchers have located a genetic marker (known as HLA-B27) associated with ankylosing spondylitis and reminiscent of the shared epitope of rheumatoid arthritis. However, this genetic marker is not a good diagnostic test for the disease because most people with the HLA-B27 marker do not have ankylosing spondylitis. Some studies suggest that women with ankylosing spondylitis are more likely to experience signs of generalized inflammation – including more fatigue, poor sense of well-being and joint swelling – than men with the condition.

Bursitis and Tendinitis

These are common conditions known as *soft tissue rheumatic syndromes*. Both conditions' symptoms include pain and inflammation in the structures and tissues around the joints. Bursitis is an irritation or inflammation of the bursa, a small sac located between bone and muscle, skin or tendon that allows for smooth movement between these structures. Tendinitis is an irritation or inflammation of the tendon, a cord that attaches muscle to bone. Bursitis and tendinitis can occur in many different joints where bursae or tendons exist, including shoulders, elbows and hips.

The pain of bursitis and tendinitis is located near joints, so some people may mistake it for arthritis. But arthritis is the inflammation of the joint itself, not the structures around the joint.

Sjögren's Syndrome

Sjögren's syndrome, which is also called sicca ("dry") syndrome, involves the salivary and lacrimal (tear-producing) glands, and leads to dry eyes and dry mouth. About 30 percent of people with rheumatoid arthritis have some evidence of Sjögren's syndrome.

The syndrome is often diagnosed through a medical history and physical examination. Some doctors may also use a variety of tests including a blood test to check the level of certain antibodies; tests to measure the dryness of eyes; a lip biopsy to examine the salivary glands; a salivary function test; or a urine test to check kidney function. Your doctor may send you to an ophthalmologist, or eye specialist, for an eye examination.

Sjögren's syndrome may be treated by a number of medications. Simple self-management strategies are also helpful, such as sipping water or chewing sugar-free gum or candies to ease dry mouth temporarily, and using over-the-counter lubricating eye drops.

Felty's Syndrome

Felty's syndrome is a form of rheumatoid arthritis that results in an enlarged spleen and a reduced number of white blood cells. Patients with Felty's syndrome are at increased risk for infections. Some physicians regard (and treat) it as a more severe form of rheumatoid arthritis.

Aggressive treatment with gold salts or methotrexate may be effective, although initially they may not seem appropriate because they may reduce the white blood cell count. Sometimes surgical removal of the spleen is required to manage Felty's syndrome.

Connective Tissue Diseases

A number of related diseases, referred to as connective tissue diseases, may be associated with arthritis, and can give the appearance of rheumatoid arthritis. Some of the more common forms of connective tissue disease are described on the following pages.

Systemic Lupus Erythematosus (Lupus)

Like rheumatoid arthritis, systemic lupus erythematosus (also called SLE or lupus) is characterized by musculoskeletal pain that is caused by inflammation and an autoimmune response. Almost all people with lupus test positive for antinuclear antibodies (ANA), but up to one-half of those with rheumatoid arthritis also have a positive ANA test.

Arthritis and skin rashes are common in people with lupus. In addition, involvement of vital organs such as the kidney or brain may occur in lupus, leading to serious complications.

Scleroderma (Systemic Sclerosis)

This disease is characterized by tightening of the skin. People with scleroderma may experience a discoloration of the hands when exposed to cold (known as Raynaud's phenomenon) – as do some people with rheumatoid arthritis. People with scleroderma may also have involvement of their internal organs, in particular the lungs, kidneys and those of the gastrointestinal track.

Polymyositis/Dermatomyositis

Polymyositis is a disease involving inflammation primarily in the muscles. The inflammation can lead to muscle weakness and permanent muscle damage. Some

Checkpoint: Your Diagnosis

Rheumatoid arthritis is not just the aches and pains of aging or of old injuries but a serious chronic illness that can affect many organs in your body. If you think you may have rheumatoid arthritis, you should see your doctor as soon as possible. Please remember that laboratory testing can be helpful, but does not provide the definitive information to make a diagnosis.

Not all doctors have extensive experience in the diagnosis and treatment of rheumatoid arthritis. Sometimes it is desirable to get a second opinion or to see a rheumatologist – a specialist in rheumatoid arthritis and related conditions, especially since controlling the joint inflammation of rheumatoid arthritis as early and as effectively as possible is important. Getting the right drug might reduce the chance of permanent damage and disability.

Remember, you are the most important member of your health-care team, but you can't do it alone. Play it safe and see a doctor.

people with polymyositis develop rashes on their hands, face or trunk, a condition referred to as dermato ("skin") myositis.

Vasculitis

Vasculitis is an inflammation of the blood vessels that can affect any organ of the body. Some people with vasculitis may have arthritis that is difficult to distinguish from rheumatoid arthritis. In rare cases, someone with rheumatoid arthritis can develop a type of vasculitis called *rheumatoid vasculitis*, and it can be difficult to determine which one is primary.

When Your Doctor Isn't Sure

Despite a medical history, physical examination and the appropriate tests, your doctor still isn't 100 percent sure whether you have rheumatoid arthritis or another type of inflammatory rheumatic disease. Should you worry?

You can probably relax. By tracking many people with inflammatory arthritis over the course of years, doctors have found that the most important matter is to identify and control the inflammation quickly. And the process for controlling inflammation is similar for most types of inflammatory arthritis, regardless of your specific diagnosis. For example, your doctor might try a nonsteroidal anti-inflammatory drug, a COX-2 specific inhibitor, or even low-dose corticosteroids (all of these drugs are discussed in detail in Chapter 11) over one to two months, even when an exact diagnosis has not been established.

Initial treatment should make you feel a lot better, have less pain and function more easily – all to your benefit. The evidence suggests that as long as your joint inflammation is controlled, the likelihood that you will develop joint damage is low.

Chapter 6

More Than Joints:
When Other Body Parts Are Affected

Although rheumatoid arthritis most commonly affects your joints, it can also target other parts of your body, including organs you may not have expected to be involved. As we mentioned in Chapter 2, rheumatoid arthritis is called a systemic disease, meaning it involves the whole body. The swelling and pain in the joints and other parts of the body result from inflammation – the primary reason you are likely to have little sense of well-being, fatigue, fevers or weight loss.

When examined carefully, many people with rheumatoid arthritis show some signs of disease affecting other organs, including the skin, eyes, mouth, lungs, heart, kidney, blood cells and spleen. Fortunately, such involvement is generally not severe and doesn't produce clinical symptoms. But sometimes, there can be important problems to address.

When other organs are affected in people with rheumatoid arthritis, an important question is whether the involvement is due to the disease, to side effects of the drugs used to treat it, or to both.

Skin

Rheumatoid nodules appear in about one-half of people with rheumatoid arthritis. The nodules are lumps of tissue that form under the skin, often over bony areas exposed to pressure (such as the fingers or the elbow). No treatment is usually necessary, unless the nodule is located in a sensitive spot, such as the spot where a person holds a pen. The nodules sometimes disappear on their own or with treatment. Interestingly, almost all people who develop nodules also have rheumatoid factor, although doctors are unsure what the connection may be, if any.

Drugs used to treat rheumatoid arthritis can also cause skin problems, such as rashes. Blue or purplish bruises sometimes appear on the skin as a result of taking corticosteroids.

Some people with RA may be affected by vasculitis (inflammation of the blood vessels), which can cause red dots to appear on the skin. This is relatively unusual, but it may be a clue that the same process is occurring in internal organs such as the lungs or kidneys. Such involvement can have serious consequences if not brought under control, although aggressive treatment with corticosteroids, methotrexate and other cytotoxic drugs (chemicals that destroy cells or prevent their multiplication) usually resolves the problem.

Eyes

People with rheumatoid arthritis who also have Sjögren's syndrome, which was mentioned in the last chapter, may experience dry eyes, which can be treated with "artificial tear" eye drops. In severe cases, a surgical procedure may help.

Some people with rheumatoid arthritis may also have an inflammation of the eyes known as *scleritis*. Doctors may treat scleritis with eye drops, as well as aggressive anti-inflammatory medications. A rare complication of scleritis is scleromalacia perforans, in which the eye may be permanently damaged by severe inflammation. If you have rheumatoid arthritis and develop eye redness that persists longer than a few days, have your eyes examined by an eye-care professional, such as an ophthalmologist, to determine if you need special treatment for scleritis. However, severe eye inflammation is rare – most people with RA will not experience this condition.

Mouth

In addition to dry eyes, people with Sjögren's syndrome may experience a severely dry mouth, because of a decrease in the body's production of saliva. As a result, they need plenty of fluids to keep their mouth moist. Good dental hygiene is a must, as bacteria tend to flourish in a dry mouth. Oral medications can help treat the dryness.

Mouth sores or oral ulcers are a frequent complication of treatment with methotrexate, and sometimes with injectable gold. Mouthwashes and lower methotrexate doses can often alleviate the problem.

Lungs

Rheumatoid arthritis can also affect the lungs. For example, it can cause *pleurisy,*

"My work day is much like anyone else's. I am a social worker and I work full time. But what I face is very different: It's hard to get out of bed on some mornings and to work buttons and zippers first thing. My hands and ankles are almost always stiff. If my ankles are swollen, I have to pick shoes that will fit. As I dress myself though, I start to loosen up and by the time I have my makeup on and leave for work, I'm able to move pretty well.

"My workday is never the same. On days when my hands are sore, I stay away from typing, and make phone calls and file papers instead. Some days I have to drive long distances to appointments. Driving isn't easy when my hands and ankles hurt. When I'm not feeling well, I get tired easily and making it through the day is hard. I'm especially tired the morning after I take my methotrexate. It would be very easy to stay home whenever I don't feel well, and I think if I started to do that, I would be home pretty often. But without my job I would never be able to afford my medical bills.

WORKING WITH RA: DAILY CHALLENGES
– DAWN MARIA DENT, PHILADELPHIA, PA

"It's hard to tell people how you feel when you don't feel well. Some people try to tell me that if I exercised more or changed my diet, my RA would go away. Even though I keep myself active and do as much as I can, at times I just can't do any more. Not everyone realizes that the pain isn't something you can just work through or talk yourself out of. Most of the people in my life treat me the same as they always did. I don't expect extra help because I have RA. But I know that without the treatments available today I wouldn't be able to function as well as I do. I don't expect people to understand what I'm going through. I just expect them to be patient with me when I'm not feeling well."

an inflammation of the lung lining that makes it painful to take a deep breath. Standard anti-inflammatory treatments for rheumatoid arthritis can alleviate this inflammation. Occasionally, people with rheumatoid arthritis may develop scarring called pulmonary fibrosis that leads to progressive shortness of breath.

Methotrexate, one of the most common RA treatments, can sometimes cause a complication known as *methotrexate lung* or *methotrexate pneumonia*. The pneumonia generally goes away when the methotrexate is stopped. Most people can safely resume taking methotrexate a few weeks later. Similar drug-induced pneumonias may occur from other, less common drugs for rheumatoid arthritis, including injectable gold and penicillamine.

Sometimes your doctor may have a hard time telling whether a lung problem results from rheumatoid arthritis or from a drug. In such cases, you and your doctor may consider additional diagnostic testing – another example of how RA and its treatments must be monitored.

Heart

Occasionally, people with rheumatoid arthritis may develop pericarditis (inflammation of the lining surrounding the heart), leading to chest pain or discomfort, and requiring direct treatment.

Kidneys

Kidneys remove waste products from the body. In some people with rheumatoid arthritis, kidney function (as measured by levels of blood urea nitrogen [BUN] or creatinine) may be reduced. Kidney problems are more likely related to side effects of RA drugs – such as cyclosporine (*Neoral*) or a nonsteroidal anti-inflammatory drug (NSAID) – than to the disease itself. If you are taking one of these drugs,

Treat Aggressively or Back Off?

The drugs used to treat rheumatoid arthritis are powerful. (See Chapter 11.) That is one reason doctors monitor patients for side effects. However, it is sometimes difficult to determine whether a complication is an effect of the disease process, during which the body's immune system turns against itself or an effect of a drug.

When possible drug side effects are noted, the tendency is to reduce dosages or stop the drugs altogether. However, in some people this approach may be a mistake.

If you face a similar situation, talk to your doctor about options. Organ involvement in some (but not all) people is more likely to be a result of the disease than a side effect of treatment. In that case, the problem should continue to be treated aggressively with the appropriate drugs.

your doctor will monitor your renal (kidney) function at periodic intervals to watch for problems.

Blood-Forming Cells

People with rheumatoid arthritis may experience a particular type of anemia, or reduction in the number of red blood cells. No special treatment is necessary for this condition, which improves as the level of inflammation in the body is brought under control.

Occasionally, people with RA develop iron-deficiency anemia, treated by iron replacement supplements. Pernicious anemia, relatively rare, can be corrected with vitamin B12 injections and/or folic acid. People with Felty's syndrome may experience a decrease in white blood cells due to an enlargement of the spleen, something treated by either drugs or, in some cases, removal of the spleen.

People with very active inflammation may have high levels of blood platelets; the levels become more normal when the inflammation is controlled. Aggressive drug treatment of rheumatoid arthritis may suppress blood cell production in the bone marrow, resulting in decreased numbers of platelets, a condition called *thrombocytopenia*. Some drugs may cause a decrease in white blood cells. Regular monitoring will identify these problems so they may be treated.

Spleen

Felty's syndrome occurs when people with rheumatoid arthritis have a reduced number of white blood cells and an enlarged spleen, suggesting that the syndrome is linked to more severe forms of rheumatoid arthritis. People with rheumatoid arthritis who develop Felty's syndrome also appear to be at increased risk for non-Hodgkin's lymphoma. So, treatments should be aggressive.

As you've learned, rheumatoid arthritis can affect many parts of the body in many ways. Regular monitoring by your physician is important, and following his treatment plan will help alleviate many problems. But what can you expect long-term from RA? In the next chapter, we'll examine long-term prognosis and how new approaches to treatment are improving that prognosis.

Chapter 7

The Long Haul:
What to Expect from RA Over Time

Chronic diseases like rheumatoid arthritis are, by definition, long-lasting. So, you may be as concerned about what will happen to you years from now as you are about what is happening in your body today. That's completely understandable, especially since living with RA can be very frustrating. You may experience periods of flare and of remission, times when your joints are stiff and painful and times when you feel fine. It's hard to know what to expect on a day-to-day basis and tough to plan ahead.

If you know other people with rheumatoid arthritis, you may be even more confused. You may meet one person with RA that is severe enough to make her quit working. You might meet another able to work and exercise. You might worry about what outcome you will experience.

All people with rheumatoid arthritis are individuals, so it's impossible to predict exactly how anyone's disease will progress over time. Nonetheless, some general guidelines can help you and your doctor establish a reasonable outline of what might happen over the course of this chronic disease.

Making a Prediction – Some Guidelines

Some factors that determine the course and severity of rheumatoid arthritis cannot be influenced by you – such as the number of joints that are involved or the level of C-reactive protein (CRP) in the blood. However, some factors you can affect, such as how quickly treatment is started and how well you adapt to the challenges of dealing with rheumatoid arthritis. Factors that influence your long-term outcome include the following:

- **The rate of disease progression.** Some

health professionals call this the "natural history" or the course that the disease takes in your body. Monitoring pain; fatigue; tenderness and swelling; level of function and disability; and the number of involved joints over several months is often the most helpful way to predict the course of disease. Lab tests may provide more information.

• **The timing of treatment.** When you first notice signs of rheumatoid arthritis, get a proper diagnosis. We cannot stress enough how important this is. The sooner treatment is started (and treatment, in almost all cases, will involve drugs that can only be prescribed by a doctor), the sooner your inflammation can be controlled. Chronic, untreated inflammation can lead to permanent, long-term damage to the joints.

• **The aggressiveness of treatment.** Early, aggressive treatment is the best tactic in fighting RA. Medications should be strong enough to bring the inflammation under control as early as possible, not just reduce the symptoms. Reducing symptoms may reduce the underlying damage to the joints and make you feel better, but aggressive treatment may prevent long-term joint damage too.

• **The ability to cope with the disease.** People who feel they are in control of chronic disease tend to have a better long-term outlook. This type of coping, or self-

efficacy, is the cornerstone of this book. Self-efficacy includes using joint-protection techniques, exercising, following your treatment plan and keeping a positive outlook.

Another Clue: Your Disease Type

Predicting the course of your disease is difficult since the progression varies from person to person. Some may find that the disease subsides after a few months, while others have inflammation and joint involvement that seems to get worse (especially if the RA is not treated). Still others travel a middle road; their disease is well controlled by medications (see box, opposite page). Below are descriptions of the three main types of rheumatoid arthritis that will help you better understand your prognosis.

Type I Disease

In the late 1960s, researchers conducted large studies involving the entire population of certain areas to see how many people met the criteria for rheumatoid arthritis. As it turned out, about two percent of the study population met the criteria. Yet, about 75 percent of those did not show evidence of rheumatoid arthritis three to five years later. And apparently many never saw a doctor about their symptoms.

It now seems likely that if a person has symptoms of rheumatoid arthritis for less than six months, chances are good that the condition will go away on its own. Doctors now better understand the early stages of RA and can better recognize this Type I rheumatoid arthritis that does not tend to progress. In fact, they may call it something other than rheumatoid arthritis – such as *inflammatory polyarthritis*. The term *rheumatoid arthritis* is now usually reserved for a more severe case of the disease.

Type II Disease

Most people who meet the criteria for rheumatoid arthritis and have experienced arthritis in symmetrical joints – both wrists, both hands, and so on – for longer than six months do not experience a spontaneous remission of their symptoms. A minority – from five percent to 20 percent – may have a mild disease course that can be controlled with less aggressive therapy (such as nonsteroidal anti-inflammatory drugs, or NSAIDs) than more

The Three Types of Rheumatoid Arthritis

	Type I	Type II	Type III
Progression	Spontaneous remission	Minimal disease progress	Serious disease progress
Percentage of people with type	5-20%	5-20%	60-90%
How is it distinguished?	Negative rheumatoid factor	Lasts more than six months; positive lab findings	Lasts more than six months; positive lab findings
Also called	Inflammatory arthritis, reactive arthritis, post-viral arthritis	Mild rheumatoid arthritis; symmetrical arthritis	Persistent inflammatory symmetrical arthritis (PISA)

severe RA. Although Type II disease is progressive, it tends to cause less severe damage to joints and often does not affect other parts of the body.

Type III Disease or PISA

Most people who have symptoms of rheumatoid arthritis for longer than six months will have what is known as *persistent inflammatory symmetrical arthritis* (PISA) or Type III disease. The most severe type of RA, it affects 60 to 90 percent of people whose disease is monitored by a doctor. The symptoms usually cannot be controlled with NSAIDs alone; stronger disease-modifying antirheumatic drugs (known as DMARDs, see Chapter 11) are needed as well to control inflammation and prevent damage.

Yes, Type III rheumatoid arthritis can have long-term consequences and require years of taking medications and monitoring by a physician. However, new information and drugs, and more aggressive treatment strategies now greatly improve the long-term outlook for this population. Because of these advances and others on the horizon, doctors believe that the joint damage that was common 20 years ago will soon be a thing of the past. People with RA now have more treatment options with fewer side effects than ever before.

Personally Speaking STORIES FROM REAL PEOPLE

"I am a registered nurse. I have had rheumatoid arthritis for several years with the usual joint pain and swelling. I had rheumatic fever as a child.

MULTIPLE COMPLICATIONS: A NURSE SPEAKS OUT
– JUDITH NAVE, ANDERSON, IN

"Approximately five years ago, I started having severe vertigo. Vomiting and barely able to stand, I went to an emergency room with a friend. All the usual tests were run, and I was given anti-nausea treatments.

"I was better after a year. Then I became blind in my right eye and my doctor referred me to a university medical center. The doctors there concluded I had rheumatoid arthritis that was affecting my right eye and my right inner ear. I am still nearly blind in my right eye. I didn't realize rheumatoid arthritis could do that to you."

Why it's Important
To See a Doctor

Clearly, the first six months of rheumatoid arthritis symptoms are telling. In some cases, the disease may go away on its own. In others, it may progress and lead to permanent damage. Why, then, is it important to see a doctor as quickly as possible if you think you may have rheumatoid arthritis? Can't you just wait it out and see if it gets better on its own?

First, it's important to see a doctor to make sure that you actually have rheumatoid arthritis, and not another disease, as mentioned in Chapter 5. An experienced doctor will consider all the evidence and make a diagnosis. Only an accurate diagnosis can assure you that you are receiving the proper treatments for your condition.

Second, you should establish some benchmark measurements during the early months to track the disease's progression. Your doctor will look for persistent joint swelling, rheumatoid factor and even early evidence of changes on X-rays.

Third, if your doctor notices evidence of progressive disease during an early visit, he or she will begin treatment to control inflammation. These drug treatments can prevent damage to joints. New and effective drugs with fewer side effects than past drugs can help you avoid serious problems and improve your long-term outlook.

Finally, nothing's wrong with seeing your doctor about a condition that may get better on its own. In fact, about one half of all visits to physicians involve such situations. In the case of rheumatoid arthritis, it's truly better to be safe than sorry.

What Changes You
Can Expect

During the 1980s, doctors realized that treatment approaches for rheumatoid arthritis did not provide a positive long-term outlook for their patients. Several rheumatology centers reported that most people with rheumatoid arthritis experienced extensive joint damage, apparent on their X-rays, in their severe decline in function and work disability, and even in a shortened life span. Something had to change. The observations led to renewed efforts to treat rheumatoid arthritis more effectively. And in fact, dramatic changes in treatment options and approaches have evolved over the last 10 years.

Doctors now have a different outlook on how rheumatoid arthritis should progress, and they monitor the progression of their patients' disease through various tests and observations. Now, doctors review changes in patients' progress as follows:

61

X-ray Changes

Over time, X-rays show joint damage in almost all people with rheumatoid arthritis who are untreated or who are not receiving aggressive treatment. In fact, about seven of 10 people develop joint changes within two years that are visible on X-rays. A magnetic resonance imaging (MRI) scan may show damage even earlier.

Although new medications can now reduce the chances of joint damage, once it occurs, it's usually irreversible. (Surgical replacement of a joint may be the only treatment option at that point, and the option is not appropriate in every case. Surgery will be discussed further in Chapter 12.) In most people, the most rapid damage occurs early, when inflammation is present – another reason to get an early diagnosis and begin drug treatment.

Changes in Function

Doctors will also measure the progress of rheumatoid arthritis by observing your ability to perform ordinary tasks, such as dressing, reaching, walking or operating household tools. Overall, more than 90 percent of people with rheumatoid arthritis report having some problems doing their usual activities. Loss of function occurs most rapidly during the first few years of the disease.

Now that treatment is more aggressive, health-care professionals have a new understanding of the biopsychosocial approach to treatment (see Chapter 1). People are more involved in managing their arthritis, so the percentage who report serious loss of function has come down. And the sooner you learn to adapt your movements or to use special aids to help you do various tasks, the sooner you will regain your freedom and ability to work and take care of yourself.

How do you cope with losing dexterity and the ability to do basic tasks? You might seek help from family members or coworkers, use special aids or devices (such as special door handle attachments), or even plan ahead to avoid excessive activity. Being creative and adapting your surroundings and activities can have a positive impact. More specific strategies will be discussed later in the book.

Work Disability

One of the more serious possible consequences of rheumatoid arthritis is work disability. Some figures show that more than one half of people with rheumatoid arthritis become unable to work after 10 years. This translates into almost one million people in the United States alone who may experience work disability

If You Face Work Disability

While many people with rheumatoid arthritis continue to work – sometimes with modifications to workspaces, schedules or even jobs – some do face the possibility of going on work disability. If you face this choice, the state-federal vocational rehabilitation program offers career counseling and vocational testing services at no cost in every state. These and other resources are listed below.

Government-Sponsored Vocational Rehabilitation Services

Most people with rheumatoid arthritis are eligible for the following services: vocational counseling and testing; job placement; assistance with resume preparation and interview skills; payment for job accommodations, training, education and travel. Check your local government listings or Web sites to find more information on vocational services in your area. Or, check the Web site of the U.S. Department of Labor, www.dol.gov, for more information on general rights and services. You can also call 866-889-5627.

Independent Living Centers

These centers provide advocacy services and programs that enable people with disabilities to live on their own. For more information, go to the Web site of Independent Living Research Utilization, a program of the Institute for Rehabilitation and Research, at www.ilru.org, or call 713-520-0232.

Job Accommodation Network

This free consulting service, funded by the Office of Disability Employment Policy, provides information about the Americans with Disabilities Act and job accommodations. The network also offers a small business self-employment service for people with disabilities. 800-526-7234 or www.dol.gov.

Disability and Business Technical Assistance Centers

Centers are available in each region of the country to advise businesses and individuals about accommodations. 800-949-4232 or www.adata.org.

The Arthritis Foundation

The Arthritis Foundation has free information about employment challenges for people with arthritis on its Web site. Visit www.arthritis.org for more information.

because of the disease. That's a serious economic problem. Yet new treatments for RA may improve the possibility of staying on the job.

Interestingly, the severity of disease does not accurately predict who will have to leave their job. Complex factors – age, occupation, the type of employer, and the amount of control over the pace of the job – determine that.

A number of resources are available to help people with disabilities continue to work (see sidebar, page 63). Since the passage of the Americans with Disabilities Act (ADA) in 1990, most employers are required by law to provide reasonable accommodations to help their employees keep working. For example, if you must stand all day to supervise employees, you may ask for job modifications from your employer.

You may be concerned about whether you can continue working. Remember, this choice should be made only after you have explored the alternatives carefully with your doctor and employer. Many job modifications cost little and can allow you to keep working without exhausting yourself or putting pressure on your joints. And many employers now allow teleworking and other alternatives to working on-site every day. While your

health condition is a private matter, you may need to discuss your diagnosis with your employer to acquire modifications or a revised work schedule. The Arthritis Foundation offers free publications to help you and your employer better understand the challenges you face. Call 800-568-4045 or log on to www.arthritis.org to get more information.

Life Span

People with rheumatoid arthritis experience many health conditions more often than the average population: infections, pulmonary disease, renal disease and gastrointestinal problems, to name a few. In addition, studies show that severe rheumatoid arthritis may decrease a person's life span by as much as 10 to 15 years compared to someone without the disease. However, many factors can determine how RA affects life span, including age of onset, the number of involved joints and ability to carry out daily activities, among others. Your approach to life with rheumatoid arthritis can have a positive impact, including taking care of your general health, not smoking, following your doctor's instructions, eating a healthy diet, getting exercise, and other good habits.

In the past five years, a number of innovative, highly effective treatments for RA (discussed in Chapter 11) became available. These treatments can reduce serious complications and enhance the life span – as well as the quality of life – of people with rheumatoid arthritis. So the outlook now is much better than ever before.

PART TWO

Join Your Health-Care Team

Chapter 8

Your Health-Care Team:
Get to Know Your Key Players

Now we have explored what rheumatoid arthritis is and how it can affect your body. Let's delve into some of the keys to the medical management of rheumatoid arthritis: What does it involve and how can you participate to get the best care and treatment possible?

Most people think of medical management in terms of drugs or medications prescribed by a doctor. You may feel that as a patient, you are a passive participant in the process. That isn't true. You are the manager of a health-care team, a collection of talented, important people who all play a position in your treatment. In a chronic disease like rheumatoid arthritis, you and your health-care team can work together to do a great deal to manage the effects of the disease.

In this chapter, we discuss the health-care professionals on your team. You may not have all of these players on your particular roster, but it's important to know what these professionals do in case you need to seek their care. In Chapter 10, we'll discuss self-management in detail to illustrate what you can do to improve your outlook. In Chapter 11, we'll review the various drugs you may take to treat your disease and its symptoms.

Who's on Your Health-Care Team?

You and your primary doctor should form a partnership to manage your arthritis. For most people with rheumatoid arthritis, that doctor is a rheumatologist. But he or she may be only one of the health-care professionals you consult during the course of your disease.

Like the disease itself, your needs may vary when it comes to your health-care team. Some people do well working with only their rheumatologist and his or her office staff, including nurses, nurse practitioners and physician assistants. Other people turn to many other health-care professionals or therapists as well.

To use an old metaphor, think of your arthritis care in terms of a play to be staged. The play should not be a one-man show, nor a cast of thousands. Instead, envision it as an ensemble production, in which each player has a particular and necessary role. In some acts, only two or three players will appear; in others, the whole cast may be on stage. Finally, you need to view yourself not only as a key player, but as the director. It will be largely up to you to decide which players can be most effective in which scenes.

Meet the Players

The composition of your health-care team depends on the particular problems or symptoms you encounter, your ability to cope with your disease and its effects, your insurance coverage, and the availability of services in your area. The following is a list and brief description of some of the health-care professionals who may play a role in your treatment.

Doctors

When we refer to doctors or physicians here, we mean medical professionals with a medical doctor (MD) degree and level of training, or in some cases, a doctor of osteopathy (DO) degree. Other medical professionals, such as doctors of podiatric medicine (DPM) and others, can be included in the category of doctors, although they specialize in certain types of care and don't provide general medical care. Doctors should fall into two subcategories: primary-care physicians, who provide general care, and specialists (or subspecialists), who have years of training beyond medical school in a specific area of medical care.

Family physicians, general practitioners and **primary-care physicians** provide medical care for adults and children with different types of arthritis and related conditions. These doctors provide the cornerstone of medical treatment for your general health and manage common additional medical problems such as high blood pressure or gastrointestinal distress. They can also help you locate a specialist. Every person should have a family physician or internist as a primary-care doctor – a specialist should not be your only doctor.

Internists specialize in internal medicine and treating adult diseases. They may

"Life is not always beautiful for my mother, Kathy. She has recently been diagnosed with rheumatoid arthritis, and it's slowly beginning to cripple her life. She has so much pain in her knees and arms and hands. It breaks my heart to see her in pain. She fears that she will be confined to a wheelchair and be deformed. If I were she, I'd fear the same things. But she is strong. She manages to raise four children and work and be an excellent mom.

MY MOTHER'S RA: AN INSPIRATION

– GABRIELLE ROGERS, GARLAND, TX

"She means so much to me. She and my father adopted me when I was an infant. I don't want her to suffer like this. Although relieving the pain and swelling at times seems hopeless, she has never pointed the finger at God. Even in the midst of pain she gives God thanks and praise: that is a true survivor. I hope that she will soon get the medicine to stop the pain she has and to help her live an easier life. She is an inspiration to me daily."

be general internists who act as primary-care physicians, or they may be subspecialists who have completed additional training in specific types of disease. A general internist provides general care to adults and often helps select subspecialists. Internists should not be confused with interns, who are doctors doing a year's training in a hospital after graduating from medical school.

Rheumatologists are internists who have additional training to treat people with arthritis or related diseases that affect the joints, muscles, bones, skin and other tissues. Most people with rheumatoid arthritis are referred to a rheumatologist at some point in their care for special assessment and treatment. Some rheumatologists may also have training in pediatrics, orthopaedics, physical medicine, sports medicine or other medical fields.

Orthopaedic surgeons or **orthopaedists** are doctors who specialize in diseases of the bone. The general area of care for specialists in orthopaedics involves mechanical problems of bones and joints, in contrast to inflammatory problems such as rheumatoid arthritis. Orthopaedists are the doctors who set fractures, repair or replace a damaged hip, knee or other joint, and treat other bone ailments. Many orthopaedists subspecialize in particular areas, such as hand surgery, sports medicine, joint replacement, etc.

When a person develops musculoskeletal pain, it is often not clear whether the problem is mechanical, inflammatory, or even based on some other type of cause, such as an infection or metabolic problem. Therefore, people with rheumatoid arthritis may be referred at first to an orthopaedic surgeon.

Pediatricians treat childhood diseases. A child who develops arthritis will see a pediatrician at first. Certain pediatricians known as ***pediatric rheumatologists*** specialize in the care of arthritis in children. These specialist pediatricians are usually located only in large cities or medical centers. A visit to such a specialist can be extremely helpful to a child with juvenile arthritis.

Physiatrists are doctors who direct physical therapy and rehabilitation programs. Comprehensive rehabilitation programs may have been more common 10 or 20 years ago when joint destruction was seen in most people with rheumatoid arthritis. Inflammation is better con-

trolled now, and this type of treatment may be less necessary for many people with rheumatoid arthritis. However, physical therapy still plays a major role in treatment for some.

Podiatrists or **chiropodists** are doctors with training in the care of the feet. These doctors may be extremely helpful to certain people with extensive disease involvement in their feet.

Psychiatrists are medical doctors who treat mental or emotional problems that need special attention. They can prescribe medications for treating the problems.

Psychologists are also trained to treat mental or emotional problems, but have a doctor of philosophy (PhD) rather than a medical degree (MD) and therefore do not prescribe medications. Psychiatrists and psychologists can be very helpful to people who have rheumatoid arthritis, as it is not uncommon that psychological issues affect their daily lives.

Other Health-Care Professionals

Some **nurses** and **nurse practitioners** are trained in arthritis and related illnesses and can assist your doctor with treatment. They can also help teach you about your treatment program and answer many of your questions or direct you to other resources for information.

Physician assistants are trained, certified and licensed to assist physicians by recording medical history and performing the physical examination, diagnosis and treatment of commonly encountered medical problems under the supervision of a licensed physician.

Physical therapists can show you exercises to help keep your muscles strong and your joints from becoming stiff. They can help you learn how to use special equipment to move better. Some physical therapists are trained to design individualized fitness programs for cardiovascular health maintenance and weight control. In general, physical therapists are concerned with larger joints – shoulders, hips and knees – and broad exercises, in contrast to occupational therapists, who are concerned with the hands and fine motor coordination.

Rehabilitation counselors can work with you to find solutions to work-related problems, such as job retraining or workplace modification.

Occupational therapists can teach you how to reduce strain on your joints while doing everyday activities. They can fit you with splints and other devices, if needed, to help reduce stress on your joints. Their role is mostly for problems with the small joints of the hands, and occasionally with arms and shoulders.

Pharmacists fill your prescriptions for medicines and can explain the actions and side effects of particular drugs. Pharmacists can tell you how different medicines work together and can answer questions about over-the-counter medications.

Social workers can help you access community resources, and they can help you find solutions to social and financial problems related to your arthritis. They may be of particular help in family situations such as helping to redistribute household responsibilities.

Getting the Most From Your Health-Care Team

Communication is the key to getting the most benefit from the health-care professionals on your team. The relationships you develop will probably be long-term ones, and will require work on both sides to develop trust and communication – much like a business partnership or a marriage. You should feel comfortable expressing your fears, asking questions you may think are stupid (but really aren't), and negotiating a treatment plan that all are satisfied with, without feeling that the health-care professionals are talking down to you or are not interested in your concerns.

There are two things to remember that will help to open (and keep open) the lines of communication. First, try to keep in mind that your doctor or therapist is only human. He or she gets tired, has headaches and experiences bad days like you do. In addition, not being able to cure someone with a chronic condition like arthritis is frustrating. Health-care professionals must take their satisfaction from seeing improvements in your condition, such as an enhanced quality of life or fewer damaged joints, rather than cures.

Second, remember that the biggest threat to a good relationship and good communication is lack of time. When time is short, there may not be enough time to fully explain things or explore options. In medical offices today, the time your doctor has to be with you is limited due to financial or insurance restraints that may be beyond his or her control. Your health professionals' anxiety about time may lead to rushed messages that you misunderstand.

Make the most of your time with each health-care professional. Be prepared ahead of time, noting questions and important changes in your condition that you wish to discuss. Remember, different health professionals can complement each other. More than one may be able to provide answers to some of your questions.

Taking P.A.R.T.

One way you can maximize the resources of your medical management team is by using a method called "Taking P.A.R.T." The technique involves preparing a list of questions or concerns before your visit, asking questions, repeating what you heard and taking action by participating as fully as you can in treatment and management decisions.

Preparing involves making and keeping your appointment, keeping a diary or journal of your symptoms and medications, and writing down questions you want answered. Make a list of all your medications, including dosages, and keep it in your wallet for easy access. Be sure to include over-the-counter medications and

Take P.A.R.T.

To get the most out of your contacts with your medical management team, remember to take P.A.R.T.:

Prepare a list of questions, concerns and symptoms.

Ask questions.

Repeat what you have heard.

Take action to reduce barriers to treatments.

supplements, too, as these can have interactions with prescription drugs. Forgetting about important questions or exact dosages of drugs is all too easy once you are in the doctor's office.

Asking your questions may take a little time, but your doctor understands these are valid concerns you have about your disease or your treatment. Bringing a prioritized list of questions to your appointment can save time and may bring up valuable information concerning your treatment.

Repeating the information or instructions you receive from your health-care professional is a great way to make sure you have heard the information correctly and that you understand it. Taking notes may also help you remember complicated instructions. Feel free to ask for written handouts or instructions.

Taking action means you are personally involved in decisions about your treatment. This step is important because it allows you to share information about your goals and preferences. Let your doctor or other health-care professionals know about your feelings, your lifestyle and your concerns. If something does not work, let him or her know so you can try something else.

Chapter 9

Keeping Tabs:
Evaluating and Monitoring Your Rheumatoid Arthritis

So far, we've learned that getting a proper diagnosis of your rheumatoid arthritis is the first, most important step. Because RA is chronic and may change over time, it's equally important to monitor the progress of your disease and regularly evaluate the effectiveness of your treatments. The goal of treatments should be to control your symptoms and to prevent permanent joint damage.

Rheumatologists measure rheumatoid arthritis disease activity in their patients through different methods, so they can determine the best individual treatment plan for each person. Even though RA varies from person to person, doctors use certain guidelines to discover how well treatments are working, or whether an additional or alternative drug is needed.

The tests and measures that doctors used to diagnose the disease are also used for ongoing evaluation and monitoring. For example, a doctor may examine a patient's joints to determine the extent of joint swelling, tenderness and range of motion, as well as the number of joints involved. In addition, X-rays, laboratory tests, functional measures and patient questionnaires provide valuable informa- tion. Patient questionnaires, which allow a person living with the disease to describe his or her symptoms and feel- ings, are a rich source of information about pain, fatigue, basic functioning, psychological distress and other conse- quences of rheumatoid arthritis.

Below are some methods and measures used to evaluate and monitor disease activ- ity, as well as any drugs' effectiveness and possible adverse effects. Although there are many different ways to evaluate and monitor rheumatoid arthritis, they can be grouped into three broad categories.

- **Measures of inflammatory activity.** Doctors measure joint tenderness and swelling, but also administer laboratory tests like sedimentation rate and C-reactive protein tests in order to measure inflammatory activity in the joints. These measures are most useful in the first few years of rheumatoid arthritis, when severe inflammation is usually present without joint damage. The results can change over time, indicating how well current drug treatments are reducing inflammation.

- **Measures of damage.** Doctors assess joint damage through examinations of mobility and joint alignment, as well as through X-rays and specialized tests of function, such as walk times, grip or button tests (i.e., how easily and quickly you can button or unbutton a garment). These measures help your doctor evaluate your quality of life, which in turn informs him about your level of joint damage. Measures of damage mostly assess changes over months to years.

- **Measures of outcome.** The biggest concern for a person with RA is: How will this disease affect me long-term? He or she is concerned with loss of function,

work disability, joint destruction and the costs associated with the disease. Experts who do long-term studies on the rheumatoid arthritis population or who sift through information such as applications for disability related to rheumatoid arthritis can predict average outcomes. This general information may be of use to you as an individual, by telling you what you may expect. But your doctor can tell you more specific information based on your unique situation, and give you advice on how to improve your outcome through treatments or lifestyle modifications.

These three types of measures do not necessarily measure the same thing. For example, joint tenderness is an effective measure of disease activity, but it is not meaningfully associated with changes that show up on X-rays. Although this may be hard to understand, it is important. Over the last 15 years evidence shows that, in some cases, measures of inflammatory activity may be stable while joint and organ damage progresses. The problem emerged as people were treated under a more cautious, less aggressive approach. The new approach to treatment – aggressive, early treatment of inflammation – may alleviate this problem.

Joint Examinations

Joint examination is one of the key ways to evaluate RA disease activity. Changes in your joint count, or the number of joints that are tender or swollen, measure the inflammation associated with rheumatoid arthritis. Joint counts help your doctor track disease progression or improvement. In addition, your doctor will probably look for any pain during motion, limitation in the motion of your joint or joint malalignment. When the structures in the joint fail to align properly, joint function is hampered.

Several different methods are used for joint counts, ranging from the simple (a rating of normal or abnormal for each joint) to the complex (four or more possible gradations for each joint). Simpler measures reveal as much as the more complex ones, and they are easier to use. The number of joints that are counted also varies, from as few as 28 to as many as 70. In long-term studies, joint counts have proved useful in assessing, monitoring and even predicting the course of rheumatoid arthritis.

X-rays and Other Imaging Techniques

X-rays (also called *radiographs*) are useful for showing specific types of changes asso-

ciated with rheumatoid arthritis. Doctors can detect narrowing of the joint space, erosion of the structures in the joint and malalignment of the joint itself. In addition, X-rays can show changes indicating osteoporosis, or thinning of the bones. The condition can be very serious and lead to painful, debilitating fractures. People with rheumatoid arthritis may be at higher risk of developing osteoporosis, and some drugs used to treat rheumatoid arthritis, such as corticosteroids, can also increase risk.

X-rays are useful for evaluating joint damage. Sometimes your doctor will take what are known as *baseline X-rays* when you are first diagnosed with rheumatoid arthritis. These are used as a basis for comparison through the years so that any changes are more easily noted.

Other, more advanced imaging techniques, such as magnetic resonance imaging (MRI) and ultrasound scanning, help doctors find evidence of inflammation before joint damage occurs. X-rays are less sensitive and primarily assess damaged joints. These newer imaging techniques may be used more often in the future for evaluating and monitoring disease activity.

Laboratory Tests

The two most widely used laboratory tests to assess inflammation are the erythrocyte

"I developed joint pain in my feet, toes, knees, hands and fingers in early November 2003. I was an ER nurse, and now I can no longer work at bedside nursing. I believed my joint pain was nothing and would go away. It worsened and I went to see a rheumatologist. X-rays showed changes related to RA. I also have problems with my urinary system and my eyes.

"I've had many difficulties. Opening doors, opening tops of containers, opening a can of soda – all of these things have become chores. When I go shopping, I have a lot of pain when I need to squat to get something on a lower shelf. My husband has to help me up because my knees hurt so much. I had to purchase a larger size shoe, and I bought ones that slip on so I don't have to tie them. I am unable to complete the blanket I was crocheting for my daughter.

RA CHALLENGES: SEEKING INFORMATION AND STAYING ACTIVE

– JAIMIE WALTON, TULSA, OK

"There are days when I cry because I don't know who to talk to or what to do. When I have very bad days, my husband comes home for lunch to help me. I feel like I have done something wrong and I'm being punished. Some days the pain is so bad, I just sit and cry. I try to keep moving. I can't lift much nor can I walk far. I go to the gym and try to swim, and I will be starting a water-exercise program to help keep my joints moving without stress. I try to walk my dog around the block every day, which helps both of us.

"I read all information about RA. I read what others with RA have to say about their lives. I will accept advice from anyone who can help me, and I will try anything that has worked for someone else."

sedimentation rate (ESR or sed rate), and C-reactive protein (CRP). As we noted before, these tests are not always abnormal in people with rheumatoid arthritis – only 60 to 70 percent of people with the disease show elevated levels. However, in people who do , the ESR and CRP can provide valuable information about disease activity over time.

Blood counts often are used to monitor adverse side effects of medications used to treat rheumatoid arthritis, such as methotrexate. The tests may be repeated periodically. For example, a low white blood cell count can indicate suppression of blood cell formation in the bone marrow. Low red blood cell counts suggest anemia and can be caused by small amounts of bleeding in the gastrointestinal tract, a possible side effect of drugs such as nonsteroidal anti-inflammatory drugs (NSAIDs).

A urinalysis, a test done on a sample of urine to determine its contents, may also be used periodically to see whether your urine contains red blood cells, protein or a variety of other abnormal substances. Again, these measures are used to monitor the effects of strong medications.

Liver function tests measure the levels of enzymes produced by the liver. The level may be elevated in people taking certain drugs for rheumatoid arthritis, including methotrexate and leflunomide (*Arava*). The tests are usually repeated every four to eight weeks.

Physical Function Measures

Physical measures of function may indicate both inflammatory activity and evidence of long-term joint damage. These measures (discussed in Chapter 3) may be repeated for comparison from one visit to another. Some of the more commonly used include measures of grip strength, walking time and manual dexterity (button test and others).

Self-Report Questionnaires

Self-report questionnaires provide a way to measure symptoms and concerns that are difficult to quantify by other, more scientific methods such as laboratory tests or X-rays. They may ask questions about pain, fatigue, loss in functional status and psychological distress. Patients can provide the best information about improvements or declines in these areas. As with other evaluative measures, doctors usually repeat questionnaires regularly to keep track of important data.

Patient questionnaires provide another avenue for your input, by asking for information that only you can provide. Take the time to fill out these questionnaires as completely, accurately and honestly as possible. Work with your doctor and other health-care professionals to develop the best treatment plan and help evaluate its effectiveness over time.

Chapter 10

Medical Management:
Effective Strategies for Treatment

Good living with rheumatoid arthritis involves much more than drugs. Nonetheless, powerful medications approved in the last decade have had the greatest impact on rheumatoid arthritis outlook in the history of the disease's treatment. Self-management, exercise and a positive outlook can make a big difference in how you feel day-to-day. Yet medications are the cornerstone of RA treatment for most people. Although there is no cure, control of inflammation to reduce pain and functional limitations is now possible in most people.

Doctors now have a much better understanding of the disease process than they did even 10 or 20 years ago. The deeper understanding of the way rheumatoid arthritis works led to the evolution of new treatment strategies with more effective medications. In addition to the introduction of new drugs, doctors now utilize older drugs in new ways, and pinpoint drug combinations that may be more helpful than using one drug at a time. These developments make the outlook for people with rheumatoid arthritis better than they have ever been.

Acute vs. Chronic Disease

In Chapter 1, we discussed some of the differences between acute and chronic diseases. Acute diseases, such a pneumonia or influenza, have a specific cause (such as a bacterium or virus), and usually have a relatively defined duration – say, a week or a month.

In an acute illness, doctors usually follow a set protocol or treatment to cure the disease. The patient is often a passive participant. He or she is only required to follow the doctor's orders and take the medications prescribed. When a person has an acute infection, doctors, nurses and other health-care professionals make most of the decisions – including which drugs to take, when to take them and what other measures are necessary. A laboratory test identifies an appropriate antibiotic, the doctor prescribes it, and the pharmacist fills the prescription. Even if the acute disease is severe and life-threatening, the outcome is known within a week or two. Many acute diseases are self-limited, such as the common cold or even a mild musculoskeletal sports injury. Drugs may cure these, hasten the recovery process or simply make a person feel better. In most cases, the person is soon back to normal.

Chronic illness is different story. Treatment cannot be regarded as a cure, but as a means to control symptoms and prevent damage. Although doctors, nurses and other health-care professionals recommend which drugs to take and when to take them, you – the patient – are the one who implements the decisions. You must make daily decisions that affect your well-being and your outcome: What to eat, whether or not to exercise, to adapt your movements or use assistive devices, to take your medications as prescribed, to seek massage therapy or other complementary pain-relief techniques. The outcome of your chronic disease, unlike acute illness, may not be known for 10 to 20 years. If you have a chronic disease like RA, you

have a great deal more control over your own management and outcome than a person with an acute illness. You become, in a sense, your own case manager.

One Drug vs. Many Drugs

Let's distinguish between diseases for which a single effective drug can be identified and diseases in which many drugs are effective. Again, many of our ideas about the treatment of diseases are derived from the treatment of an infectious disease. In an infectious disease, we sometimes forget that although a person may appear to be cured by taking an antibiotic, the target of the antibiotic is not the person, but rather a specific microorganism. In this situation, a drug that works in one person is likely to work equally well in other people with the same infection, although some people may have allergic reactions and need an alternative treatment. It's usually possible to identify the most effective drug for a given infection, because the same microorganism is involved in each case.

People with rheumatoid arthritis are complex and differ from one another in genetic makeup, levels of nutrition, age, lifestyle, background and many other factors that may affect the choice of a drug. So no single best drug works for all people, although certain drugs work better in more people than other drugs. Naming the best drug for all people with rheumatoid arthritis is a little like trying to name the best flavor of ice cream for all people: One flavor might be preferred by most people, but there will always be some people who like another flavor better.

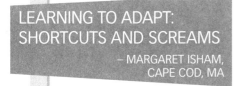

Personally Speaking STORIES FROM REAL PEOPLE

"After being diagnosed three years ago (following a diagnosis of Lyme disease the year before), I've had some good times and some bad ones. The past few months have been hard. I am an otherwise healthy, 47-year-old teacher, but the RA makes me really tired and dependent on others to do certain tasks. I'm afraid that I may fall getting out of the bath, and I'm crabby about doing chores like the dishes, because it hurts. (Isn't that a great excuse for skipping the housework?!)

"I'm a very independent single mother with a wonderful boyfriend, and when he tries to help me out more than I like, I say, 'No, I am fine,' which drives him crazy because it is obvious that I am not. So, I am learning to accept more help and not be so independent. That is very hard for me.

LEARNING TO ADAPT: SHORTCUTS AND SCREAMS
– MARGARET ISHAM, CAPE COD, MA

"I have been learning to adapt: I try different types of toothpaste to find one that's easy to squeeze out of the tube. Once a pill bottle is open, I move the whole contents to a baggie because the bottles are hard to open. I cut packages, bags of cat food and kitty litter open instead of trying to rip them.

"I have actually screamed at the RA once or twice when I am alone in the house and feeling frustrated. I feel a bit crazy because normally I'm a mild-mannered, easy-going person who never screams. But it's good to let it out. I have had to give up the treadmill and weight lifting, but when I can, I do Pilates and yoga. Next will be swimming although I am not someone who likes swimming.

"I sometimes worry about my future. I do not want to be a bed-ridden old hag, and some days I sure feel like one. I certainly have needed to become quieter and more sedate. No more wild and crazy nights out!"

The Old Approach to Medical Management

The medical approach to treating rheumatoid arthritis, as well as other chronic diseases, is based on a principle to "do no harm." That is, the treatment prescribed should not be worse than the disease itself. This remains a valid principle in any type of medical care – as long as the judgment of what is harmful is based on a realistic assessment of how harmful the disease might be.

When using the old approach, sometimes called the *pyramid approach*, doctors were concerned that many of the drugs might be more harmful to people than the rheumatoid arthritis. Doctors started at the base of a treatment pyramid with first-line drugs, such as nonsteroidal anti-inflammatory drugs (NSAIDs) or salicylates (the most common of which is aspirin), along with simple measures such as patient education and physical therapy. If these medicines did not control the disease, doctors then moved up the pyramid to the more powerful disease-modifying antirheumatic drugs (DMARDs) and immunosuppressive drugs. Progressing up the pyramid could take quite a while, because the effectiveness of many of the drugs cannot be determined immediately; it can sometimes take several months.

The problem with applying this approach to rheumatoid arthritis was that, in the past, doctors did not have a complete understanding of the disease process or the amount of joint damage that could result in the first few years. Research has since shown that joint damage probably begins in the first two years of persistent arthritis. Once these factors were understood, the strategy of treatment changed and doctors began prescribing more powerful medicines earlier in the course of the disease.

Another problem with the old approach to treatment is that some of the older drugs, such as gold injections and penicillamine, have a much higher likelihood of side effects than newer drugs, such as the biologic drugs or methotrexate. And the newer drugs have allowed more aggressive approaches at an earlier stage of the disease, when joint damage may still be prevented.

The New Approach: A Preventive Strategy

Doctors now prescribe powerful drugs early in the disease course in an effort to control inflammation and prevent damage to joints. This new approach is similar to the early, aggressive treatment of high blood pressure to prevent long-term damage to the heart and blood vessels. Rheumatoid arthritis can lead to severe long-term outcomes. By recognizing and even emphasizing the possible damage to the body, doctors, other health professionals, patients, friends and families can act to prevent these consequences.

This approach to prevention has made a big difference in treating cardiovascular disease and is now making one in treating rheumatoid arthritis. For most people with RA, rheumatologists use combinations of available drugs to find the right treatment program for each individual. In fact, most people must take at least two drugs to adequately control disease, and many people take three or four drugs.

Is This New Approach Safe?

The old approach to treating rheumatoid arthritis was slow and often produced disappointing results. In addition, some of the drugs thought to be less harmful actually had fairly severe side effects and led to poor long-term outcomes. Many people with rheumatoid arthritis had lost hope. What about the new approach? Is it really more effective? And are these new drugs safe?

Evidence is still incomplete about the

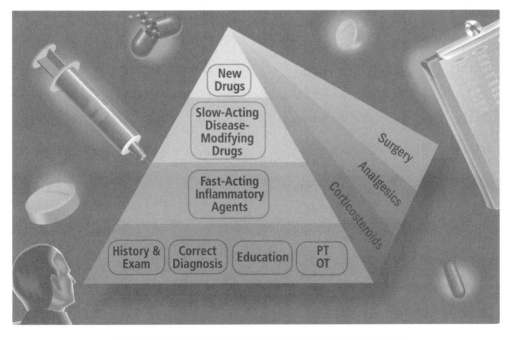

THE TRADITIONAL OR "PYRAMID" APPROACH TO TREATMENT

long-term – and possibly toxic – effects of combining several drugs – especially the powerful, disease-modifying ones – to treat rheumatoid arthritis. However, research studies indicate that combinations of drugs are no more likely to cause side effects than drugs taken individually. Aggressive therapy, including drug combinations, has the potential to minimize the kind of joint damage that once occurred during the early years of disease. Of course, different people have different responses to the medications. Some individuals will do just fine with a conservative approach, but others will need more aggressive treatment strategies.

The issue is really not so much "Is my disease so bad that I need the aggressive treatment?" but rather, "Can I be better off in five years with aggressive treatment?" The "side effects" of rheumatoid arthritis itself are considerably worse than the side effects of many new drugs. Doctors have refined the drug dosages necessary to achieve good results and keep side effects in mind as they prescribe medications.

What You Can Do

You play a vital role in your RA treatment. Learn about the drugs your doctor prescribes: how they work, the benefits and the potential side effects. Keep track of how your drugs seem to be working and what side effects you have, and share this information with your doctor during your appointments. Alert your doctor early to signs of a particular side effect so your medication can be reduced or changed. Also, take your medication according to the doctor's instructions because this can help prevent or minimize side effects.

On the following three pages, you'll find worksheets to help you prepare for each doctor's visit, to talk openly with your doctor during the visit, and to better understand your medications and how to take them. Feel free to photocopy these worksheets and use them for each new doctor's visit.

Rheumatoid arthritis takes a different course in every person with the disease. So your needs and reactions to the drugs may differ from those of others. But your needs and reactions are what your doctor will consider first when developing or changing your treatment program.

Stopping Drug Treatment

Your medications may make you feel greatly improved. You may even be tempted, at certain points, to discontinue drug therapy because you feel so good. Stopping the therapy may be all right for a few weeks or even months. However, in most patients, a relapse is almost inevitable, usually within several weeks or months. In addition, getting the disease back under control will often be more difficult. So, although it may be hard for you to take drugs when the disease isn't evident, most experts recommend this approach. The best strategy is to keep things as normal as possible to prevent damage, which includes treatment even when your symptoms disappear.

In the next chapter, we'll discuss the many drugs available to treat rheumatoid arthritis, including new medications that have changed the course of RA treatment.

WORKSHEET: "Ask the Doctor"

Complete this before the visit:

1. What is the main reason I am going to the doctor?

   _____

   _____

2. Is there anything else that concerns me about my health or treatment (e.g., effect of RA on work, family or mood; problems following the recommended treatment plan)? _____Yes _____No
   If so, what?

   _____

3. What do I want the doctor to do today?

   _____

   _____

4. The symptoms that bother me the most are ... (What? Where? When did they start? Do they change over time? How long do they last?). NOTE: Bring copies of any completed self-monitoring forms/diaries.

   _____

   _____

5. What medications (prescriptions and over-the-counter) am I taking regularly? (List name(s) and dosage, or take the bottles to your appointment.)

   _____

   _____

6. What are my goals for treatment (what I want or expect to get out of treatment)?

   _____

   _____

7. Prepare and prioritize a list of questions to give the doctor early in the visit.

   _____

   _____

8. Do I need Medicare, Medicaid or other insurance cards/forms today?
   _____Yes _____No

WORKSHEET: "Ask the Doctor"

Questions to ask your doctor during the visit:

1. What is happening to me? How is my RA likely to affect me?

   _____

   _____

2. What are the results of my tests, and what do they mean? May I have a copy of the results?

   _____

3. Why do I need the lab tests or X-rays that you are recommending today?

   _____

4. Are there any risks from these tests?

   _____

5. When should I call for the results?

   _____

6. What should I do at home (diet, activity, treatment options, special instructions, medications, precautions, etc.)?

   _____

a. What are the benefits, costs and drawbacks for each treatment option?

   _____

b. How and how often do I do the treatment?

   _____

7. When should I call if my condition doesn't improve and the treatment doesn't seem to be working? What symptoms warrant my calling before my next scheduled visit?

   _____

8. When should I return for another visit?

   _____

WORKSHEET: "Ask the Doctor"

Medication questions:

1. What is the name of the drug? _____

2. What are the purpose and benefits of the drug? _____

3. How quickly does it work? How long should I take the drug?
   _____

4. What are the possible side effects or drawbacks to the drug?
   _____

a. When should I contact you about side effects? _____

b. What can I do to prevent or deal with the side effects or drawbacks?
   _____

5. Is it all right to take the drug with other drugs (such as cold, sinus, allergy, pain medicines) I am taking? _____Yes _____No
   If not, what drugs should I avoid? _____

6. When is the best time to take the drug? Before, with or after meals?
   _____

7. What should I do if I forget to take my medicine?
   _____

8. Are there any changes I should make in my diet? _____Yes _____No
   If so, what? _____

a. Can I drink alcohol while taking this drug? _____Yes _____No

b. Are there any other restrictions? _____Yes _____No
   If so, what? _____

9. Should I avoid driving while taking this drug? _____Yes _____No

10. Is a generic drug available? If so, is generic as effective? _____Yes _____No

Chapter 11

Aggressive Therapy:
Drugs to Treat Rheumatoid Arthritis

Good living with rheumatoid arthritis involves many self-management activities, many of which focus on diet, exercise and coping with stress. But the most important component of treatment is drugs. A number of new, effective drugs have emerged to change the face of RA treatment. In this chapter, we'll go over categories of drugs, medications and other drug-related issues.

You play an important role in this area of your RA treatment. Although only your doctor can prescribe many of the drugs included in this chapter, you must work hard to take them properly, regularly and according to your doctor's instructions. You must keep track of the other drugs, herbs, and supplements you take – even for conditions other than your arthritis, such as high blood pressure, headaches, or sleep problems. You must check the prescriptions your pharmacist dispenses to make sure you are getting the correct medicine and keep track of changes in your drug insurance coverage. Most important, you must stay informed about drugs for rheumatoid arthritis.

This chapter will provide a good basis for your RA drug education. At the end of this book, you will find more resources – including directions for contacting the Arthritis Foundation chapter in your area – that can help you get updated information about drug treatments.

Prescription vs. Over-the-Counter Drugs

Drugs can be categorized in many ways, but the most basic distinction is this: Some drugs are available only by prescription and others are available over the counter. A prescription medication is one that requires a doctor's written order – or phone call to the pharmacy. Over-the-counter, or OTC, drugs can be purchased without a prescription, either at drugstores, supermarkets, convenience stores, or over the Internet. But OTC drugs are serious medications, too. Many OTC drugs can be prescribed in stronger doses.

OTC arthritis medications include the analgesic medication acetaminophen (*Tylenol*) and four nonsteroidal anti-inflammatory drugs (NSAIDs) – ibuprofen (*Advil, Motrin*), naproxen sodium (*Aleve*), ketoprofen (*Orudis KT*) and aspirin (*Bayer, Bufferin*). Although these drugs come in many formulations and in combination with other ingredients (such as caffeine to speed pain relief, antihistamines to cause drowsiness, or a diuretic to ease menstrual bloating) they are the only over-the-counter medications that ease pain. They often come in generic store brands as well.

Prescription drugs are becoming increasingly available over the counter, usually in lower doses. Getting a medication has never been more convenient and less expensive. You don't need an appointment with a physician if all you need is something to ease the pain of an occasional headache or muscle strain. But people are more likely than ever to medicate themselves with readily available drugs without consulting their doctor. A 2004 report at the annual American Gastroenterological Association meeting suggested that many people take more OTC pain relievers than is necessary or safe, increasing the risk of serious stomach problems.

You may think that any drug you can buy over the counter is safe to use as you please, adjusting the dosage as you see fit. This is not true. It's important to follow the directions on the label exactly. You also should contact your doctor promptly if you suspect an adverse reaction or side effect to taking OTC drugs, or if symptoms don't improve.

OTC drugs may contain similar (or identical) active ingredients to the prescription drugs you take. So taking an over-the-counter medication such as *Advil* along with your prescription of *Motrin* may lead to an overdose. Tell your doctor about all the medications you take, including over-the-counter medicines. Fortunately, most OTC medications have new labels that help you understand the active ingredients inside and how to take them properly. OTC medications that don't have the labels yet will soon be required by law to have them.

In the coming sections, we'll look more closely at the general categories of drugs used to treat rheumatoid arthritis. Most of these drugs are available by a doctor's prescription only. At the end of the chapter, we provide a drug chart that you can use to look up information about each of the drugs.

Nonsteroidal Anti-Inflammatory Drugs (NSAIDs)

Nonsteroidal anti-inflammatory drugs or NSAIDs are drugs similar to aspirin that can reduce inflammation. By doing so, they also relieve pain. There are three generations of these drugs: The first is aspirin, which taken regularly in non-coated form, is often irritating to the stomach. The second generation is other forms of aspirin (such as enteric-coated aspirin – aspirin coated with a substance that allows it to pass through the stomach into the small intestine before it is released; and zero-order release aspirin, or aspirin that steadily releases for a given period) and drugs such as ibuprofen (*Motrin, Advil*), naproxen (*Naprosyn, Aleve*), indomethacin (*Indocin*) and others. These are often as effective as aspirin, but with less irritation to the stomach. Most recently, a third generation of NSAIDs known as COX-2 inhibitors has been developed. As of press time, celecoxib (*Celebrex*) is the only COX-2 on the market. COX-2s were designed to offer greater safety from gastrointestinal problems. However, they carry a risk of heart attack, stroke, blood clot or severe skin reactions. Two other COX-2s originally available were voluntarily pulled from the market because of the risks. Always talk to your doctor for the latest information on COX-2s.

NSAIDs reduce (and sometimes even eliminate) inflammation, lessening pain in people with rheumatoid arthritis. Joint inflammation results from the production of chemicals called *cytokines*, which, in turn, stimulate a subgroup of chemicals called *prostaglandins*. A primary action of NSAIDs is to inhibit production of prostaglandins, which in turn reduces the inflammation and pain associated with rheumatoid arthritis.

As we discussed in Chapter 2, inflammation normally serves to protect the body from invasion by an infection or bacterium and helps heal wounds such as a cut or fracture. Prostaglandins and cytokines are not in the body to be harmful, but to protect us. When inflammation has accomplished its mission, complex control mechanisms should stop the production of the chemicals. But in people with RA, prostaglandins and cytokines are produced when they shouldn't be, leading to inflammation, pain and long-term damage.

NSAIDs and Stomach Distress

In addition to their role in inflammation, prostaglandins perform necessary functions in certain tissues and organs. Prostaglandins help protect the lining of the stomach from acid, which can eat away at the stomach and cause bleeding or a hole in the stomach called an *ulcer*. Ulcers can be very serious. Because NSAIDs reduce the production of prostaglandins, they may cause stomach irritation and undesirable gastrointestinal side effects.

Prostaglandins also aid in removal of fluid from the kidneys, maintain a balance of competing chemicals in the brain, and promote normal blood clotting in platelets. That's why NSAIDs may cause problems with kidney function, such as fluid retention; with central nervous system function, such as headaches and feeling "spacey"; or interfere with normal blood clotting. The possibility of bleeding is the reason surgeons ask patients to stop taking NSAIDs for a week or two prior to any surgery. Some of the newer NSAIDs cause fewer of these problems. We'll discuss those new treatments later in the section.

Aspirin: The Classic NSAID

Aspirin has been used as a medicine since ancient times. Long ago, people realized that eating the bark of the willow tree, or drinking a tea brewed from the bark, could help treat pain and certain illnesses. In the late 19th century, the active chemical in willow bark (called salicylate) was synthesized as a pill: the birth of modern aspirin.

Aspirin remains an effective drug for relief of inflammation and pain. However, plain aspirin is too irritating to the stomach for long-term use in the high quantities needed for treating rheumatoid arthritis. Newer forms of aspirin including Ascriptin (aspirin mixed with *Maalox*), enteric-coated aspirin (*Ecotrin*) and zero-order release aspirin (*ZORprin*) were created. These drugs cause much lower levels of stomach irritation. Even when aspirin is not absorbed in the stomach (for instance, when it is given as a suppository through the rectum or as a zero-order release aspirin absorbed in the small intestine), some stomach irritation occurs, indicating that general systemic effects of aspirin lead to stomach irritation.

Past studies have shown that the newer, less irritating forms of aspirin were favored by more people with rheumatoid arthritis than any of the other NSAIDs available before 1990. There is still a place for aspirin and its spin-offs in the treatment of certain people with rheumatoid arthritis.

Other Traditional NSAIDs

Beginning in the 1970s, a number of other NSAIDs were developed by the pharmaceutical industry and are now widely used. Indomethacin (*Indocin*) and ibuprofen (*Motrin, Advil, Nuprin*) were among the first developed. (Ibuprofen is available over the counter in lower doses.) These anti-inflammatory drugs did not have the same chemical composition as aspirin, and many people found them easier to take. Nonetheless, these NSAIDs carried with them the same potential side effects as aspirin – irritation of the stomach, interference with the kidneys' removal of fluid, imbalance in the central nervous system and reduced blood clotting. But these side effects occurred less often than they did with aspirin.

Indomethacin is usually not very helpful to most people with rheumatoid arthritis, although a few people experience great benefit. Indomethacin may cause unacceptable headaches and "spacey" feelings in more people than any other NSAID. But everyone is different (one of the recurring themes of this book); if only two percent of people with rheumatoid arthritis benefit from indomethacin use, for those few, the drug is well worth trying.

Ibuprofen was the first major alternative to aspirin and was launched with great fanfare. Many people who take ibuprofen experience as much pain relief as with aspirin, but have less gastrointestinal discomfort. In addition, there is a lower risk of severe gastrointestinal irritation and other side effects than with aspirin. Ibuprofen is the most widely used NSAID, particularly since 1992 when it became available over the counter as *Advil, Nuprin, Motrin* or *Mediprin*. However, the nonprescription 200-mg dose is often not sufficient for people with rheumatoid arthritis, although it may be quite effective for a relatively minor trauma such as a strained muscle. People with rheumatoid arthritis often need 400, 600 or even 800 mg of ibuprofen several times a day to gain effective pain relief.

One drawback to ibuprofen, aspirin and other traditional NSAIDs is that they must be taken at least three or four times per day to give people the best benefit because their effects only last for a few hours. This problem led scientists to develop longer-acting NSAIDs, which only need to be taken twice or even once per day. Some of the more widely used long-acting NSAIDs include naproxen (*Naprosyn*), which is available in doses of 250, 375 and 500 mg, and is also available without a prescription as *Aleve* in a dose of

99

220 mg. Other twice-a-day compounds include nabumetone (*Relafen*), ketoprofen (*Orudis, Oruvail*) and diclofenac (*Voltaren*). Indomethacin also comes in a slow release form for twice daily usage (*Indocin SR*). Some of the once-a-day NSAIDs include piroxicam (*Feldene*) and oxaprozin (*Daypro*). Although these newer NSAIDs are taken less frequently, they still have the same potential gastrointestinal side effects of NSAIDs.

The Gastrointestinal Dilemma

Doctors recognized the problem of gastrointestinal irritation caused by NSAIDs in the 1980s. Several types of research studies indicated that every year about one of every 50 to 100 people who took NSAIDs regularly experienced a major gastrointestinal event, such as bleeding ulcer or perforation, leading to hospitalization. That may not sound like a lot of people, but if millions of people take these drugs, then thousands could expect to have serious side effects from the use of NSAIDs.

A person might experience an acute problem resulting from NSAIDs such as internal bleeding, a hole or perforation, or an obstruction in the stomach without any warning signs or symptoms such as pain, nausea or heartburn. Other people may have many symptoms and never experience a serious gastrointestinal event. Although patients and doctors respond primarily to symptoms – that is, reports of heartburn or stomach pain – the major reason to be concerned about the gastrointestinal tract may not be pain, but risk of a serious event. The risk increases substantially in people over age 75, those with a previous history of gastrointestinal events and those with more active, severe joint disease.

The risk prevents many people from taking traditional NSAIDs. Now that disease-modifying antirheumatic drugs (DMARDs) are used early in the course of the disease, as we discussed in Chapter 10, NSAIDs are no longer regarded as the mainstay of the treatment. Yet more than 60 percent of RA patients continue to take these drugs, more for pain relief than for their anti-inflammatory activity. NSAIDs are widely used for treating other rheumatic conditions, including osteoarthritis, tendinitis and bursitis. Because they are useful, widely used drugs, here are four strategies to help reduce gastrointestinal side effects of NSAIDs:

• **Combine NSAIDs with antacid drugs.** The first strategy involves the addition of drugs that might protect the lining of the stomach. One of the early attempts was a combination of aspirin and Maalox (*Ascriptin*), which many people found to cause less gastrointestinal irritation than plain aspirin. However, there was still a substantial rate of gastrointestinal ulcers and irritation – apparently because the aspirin's chemical properties still irritated the stomach. So, the strategy helped alleviate some symptoms, but it did not necessarily reduce the risk of serious events.

• **Add H2 blockers.** During the 1970s, a new class of compounds was developed called H2 blockers. These agents included cimetidine (*Tagamet*), famotidine (*Pepcid*), ranitidine (*Zantac*) and nizatidine (*Axid*). Now, many of these drugs are available over the counter as well as in prescription form. H2 blockers act by blocking receptors in the stomach that lead to the production of acid. The net result is less acid production. The drugs reduce some of the gastrointestinal irritation associated with NSAIDs, but the protection is far from complete.

• **Combine with synthetic prostaglandins.** Researchers have developed a pill that contains a synthetic prostaglandin called misoprostol (*Cytotec*). When taken with an NSAID, it helps to protect the stomach from irritation. Another drug that contains diclofenac (*Voltaren*) coated with misoprostol (*Arthrotec*) is another option. Arthrotec can be taken twice per day, and many

people have found it effective.

• **Add proton pump inhibitors.** A recently introduced class of gastrointestinal compounds known as proton pump inhibitors often provides even more effective relief than H2 blockers. Examples include omeprazole (*Prilosec*) (also now available in an over-the-counter dosage), lansoprazole (*Prevacid*) and esomaprazole magnesium (*Nexium*). Studies have documented that proton pump inhibitors can protect the stomach against the gastrointestinal side effects associated with NSAIDs, blocking the secretion of acid into the stomach more effectively than H2 blockers.

COX-2 – Specific Inhibitors

During the 1990s, scientists discovered that two types of enzymes called cyclooxygenase enzymes, or COX enzymes, lead to the synthesis of prostaglandins. Cyclooxygenase-1 (COX-1) is associated with many of the "healthy" functions of prostaglandins, such as protecting the lining of the stomach, helping to remove fluids, maintaining balance in the central nervous system and promoting blood clotting. Cyclooxygenase-2 (COX-2) is associated with other functions of prostaglandins, including the inflammatory response.

In theory, a drug that inhibits COX-2 but not COX-1 would be able to inhibit the inflammatory response that occurs in rheumatoid arthritis without having the undesirable effects of some of the traditional NSAIDs, particularly the possibility of irritating the stomach and causing gastrointestinal problems such as bleeding and perforation of the stomach. But there is now new concern that COX-2 drugs, because they do not inhibit COX-1, do not provide the protection against cardiovascular problems (heart attacks and strokes) that regular NSAIDs (such as low-dose aspirin, a common preventive treatment for cardiovascular disease) provide. In fact, they increase the risk of heart attack, stroke, blood clot or severe skin reactions. Long-term studies to evaluate the cardiovascular and other risks associated with COX-2 drugs are underway. It may also take years of study before doctors know whether COX-2 drugs safely prevent serious gastrointestinal complications.

One selective COX-2 inhibitor is available on the market: celecoxib (*Celebrex*). At one time, three COX-2s were available, including celocoib (*Celebrex*), rofecoxib (*Vioxx*) and valdecoxib (*Bextra*). As of press time, only celecoxib (*Celebrex*) remains available.

Rofecoxib (*Vioxx*) was pulled from the market by its manufacturer in September 2004, which cited increased risk of heart attack and stroke. In April 2005, Valdecoib (*Bextra*) was also pulled from the market by its manufacturer at the urg-ing of the Federal Drug Administration. It was voluntarily pulled because of possible risk of heart attack, stroke and reports of severe skin reactions.

Talk with your doctor to get the latest information about COX-2s.

Do NSAIDs Have a Role in the Future of RA Treatment?

Doctors are now reassessing the role of NSAIDs in rheumatoid arthritis treatment. Previously they felt that NSAIDs should be used in all RA patients as the first line of therapy. However, now that powerful new disease-modifying antirheumatic drugs (DMARDs) are available, some people may not need NSAIDs.

Many doctors are now using NSAIDs primarily for their analgesic (pain-relieving) properties. The drugs are able to relieve pain in addition to relieving inflammation. Very few people with rheumatoid arthritis are treated with NSAIDs alone because NSAIDs alone are not sufficient to block the progression of joint destruction and functional disability. Instead, they may be used in combination with DMARDs to to control pain and inflammation.

Analgesics

Analgesic drugs relieve pain without necessarily having an effect on inflammation.

The prototype drug in this class is acetaminophen (*Tylenol*), which may be combined with other pain-relieving drugs such as codeine. Acetaminophen is the drug that the American College of Rheumatology recommends as the first response to general arthritis pain. Another widely used analgesic drug is propoxyphene (*Darvon*). In addition, there are stronger narcotic analgesic drugs such as meperidine (*Demerol*), morphine, and compounds such as *Percocet, Percodan, Vicodin*, and others.

Analgesic drugs relieve pain because they act on the brain or the central nervous system, where pain is perceived. As discussed in Chapter 2, rheumatoid arthritis pain is best relieved by controlling inflammation through the use of anti-inflammatory drugs. However, in certain patients at certain times – and in people who have painful joints as a result of joint damage, but no longer have active inflammation – it is often helpful to use analgesic drugs specifically to relieve pain. In addition, they may need analgesics to relieve other painful problems, such as a tooth extraction or menstrual cramps.

Pain: It's All in Your Head
Sometimes people confronted with severe pain may ask, "Is all of this pain in my head?" The correct answer is yes, sort of. All pain is experienced in the head, although it may reflect problems in an arm or leg. Inflammation in the joints of your hands may send signals that something is wrong through your central nervous system to your brain, which interprets the signals and responds with pain. If you have a fractured leg that needs to be manipulated, you may be given anesthesia and put to sleep, at which point you feel no more pain. The perception of pain can be more or less depending, in part, on how the brain interprets the signals it receives.

Of course, sometimes pain cannot be explained by inflammation or structural changes. Thus common form of musculoskeletal pain is experienced by people who have fibromyalgia. People with rheumatoid arthritis may also have fibromyalgia, as discussed in Chapter 5, and may require additional therapy to treat these problems.

Acetaminophen
The most widely used analgesic drug in the United States is acetaminophen (*Tylenol*), also known as paracetamol (*Panadol*) in Europe. It is available over the counter in low doses and under various brand names. Acetaminophen may be a good substitute for NSAIDs in some

people when it comes to reducing fever or relieving pain. However, it only slightly relieves inflammation, one of the primary actions of aspirin. So although you can substitute acetaminophen for an aspirin when you have a headache or a toothache, you cannot substitute acetaminophen for aspirin to relieve the inflammation of rheumatoid arthritis.

Acetaminophen is now recommended as the first drug to be used for osteoarthritis, which in effect is what a person with rheumatoid arthritis who has damaged joints may be experiencing. So acetaminophen may be helpful when pain is not the result of inflammation but of long-term damage to joints resulting from rheumatoid arthritis.

Acetaminophen is often combined with a narcotic. Most frequently it is mixed with codeine as *Tylenol* #1, 2, 3 or 4, containing 15, 30, 45 and 60 mg of codeine, respectively. This combination is used by doctors for conditions that may cause pain beyond the rheumatoid arthritis or to "tide you over" during a flare of disease activity. Acetaminophen as a single drug or as a compound is usually not an effective long-term drug to be used for treating rheumatoid arthritis.

Narcotic Analgesics

A number of narcotic analgesic drugs are used as pain relievers for people with rheumatoid arthritis. In general, these drugs relieve pain more effectively than anti-inflammatory drugs or non-narcotic analgesic drugs. They include codeine, meperidine (*Demerol*), propoxyphene (*Darvon*), morphine, oxycodone, hydrocodone and a newer drug, tramadol (*Ultram*), which can also be mixed with acetaminophen (*Ultracet*). These drugs are often used in combination with acetaminophen and other drugs.

A rule of thumb in treating rheumatoid arthritis or other rheumatic diseases has been to avoid the use of narcotic drugs. Although it is true that one should think twice about the use of narcotic drugs, this position has been modified as the position about prednisone and other drugs has been modified. Physicians now believe that many people may benefit from the judicious use of narcotic drugs. Although dependence is a danger, studies show that people who experience severe pain are unlikely to become addicted unlike people who have no pain but take narcotic drugs for other types of effects on the brain, or for pleasure.

Doctors have different views of the use of narcotic drugs. In general, studies show that doctors tend to underestimate pain experienced by patients. To the patient's frustration, this can lead to under-medication.

The Narcotics Debate

Some doctors would never prescribe narcotics for RA pain, while others argue that they can be appropriate treatments for pain. If pain relief is not achieved with NSAIDs, COX-2 drugs, or other treatments, some doctors will consider narcotics.

The decision requires patient counseling on dependency and expected side effects. Some physicians require patients to sign a contract that outlines appropriate use of the drugs and the physician's expectations regarding ongoing use. Here are what many doctors view as central issues in the debate:

Advantages:

- Narcotics are the most effective available medications for managing chronic pain.

- The majority of patients don't need narcotics. But those that do should have the option for a trial period.

- The addiction rate from narcotics is one percent. Addiction (compulsive, self-destructive use) is not the same as dependence (withdrawal symptoms if the drug is stopped abruptly).

- Less pain results in better functioning.

Disadvantages:

- When you use narcotics, you are treating pain solely as a symptom, without necessarily eliminating the factors that cause it. Narcotics should be used only in the context of a thorough medical management program.

- Dependence is an expected result of treatment.

- Narcotics will dull pain, but not eliminate it. In other words, they are not a cure for arthritis.

- Tolerance to narcotics occurs after a time – from months to years – so that increasing the dosage is necessary to maintain the same level of response.

- Narcotics have side effects such as mental fuzziness, constipation, nausea, drowsiness and itching that add to the side effects of other medications.

If you feel that your pain is not sufficiently managed by the drugs you are currently taking, talk to your doctor about other options. For more information, read *The Arthritis Foundation's Guide to Pain Management,* available by calling 800-283-7800 or at www.arthritis.org.

Questionnaires that score pain levels have been very helpful in documenting pain severity from a patient's perspective, and many doctors use these measures to judge the need for additional pain relief. Pain management is now one of the fastest growing segments of medical treatment, and medical schools now emphasize pain management. In some cities, special pain centers and pain clinics focus on treating pain, especially in patients with chronic illnesses.

A number of narcotic compounds treat pain. The drugs are most effective for treating painful flares or pain resulting from a fracture or other severe acute events. These drugs include *Percodan*, *Percocet* and *Lortab*. Narcotic compounds can also be given in the form of a patch worn on the skin, such as the *Duragesic* patch. This may be helpful when a person experiences acute pain, for instance, in the case of a compression spine fracture, which heals over weeks to months without long-term consequences.

One simple analgesic drug that has been used extensively is propoxyphene (*Darvon*). The drug's pain relief is comparable to acetaminophen. However, as with all drugs, some people find propoxyphene more effective than acetaminophen, and some do not.

Corticosteroids

Probably no drugs used in the treatment of rheumatoid arthritis, or even in clinical medicine, evoke more controversy than this class. Corticosteroids are a group of life-sustaining and anti-inflammatory hormones that are produced naturally by the adrenal gland, an internal organ situated above the kidney. They help support the circulatory system and regulate body functions. All of us make about 25 mg to 35 mg of cortisol (our naturally occurring corticosteroid) each day to support vital body functions.

When cortisone, a synthetic form of corticosteroids, was first given to people with rheumatoid arthritis in 1948, doctors viewed it as miracle drug and perhaps even a cure. Unfortunately, cortisone or prednisone – the most commonly used chemical form of cortisone and one of the most important drugs in the treatment of rheumatoid arthritis – caused many serious side effects that often became worse than the disease itself.

From the 1950s through the 1980s, doctors recommended that cortisone or prednisone not be used for rheumatoid arthritis, except for treating the most severe complications. However, over the last 15 years doctors have recognized that low doses of cortisone, such as 5 mg of prednisone or less, can be taken over long periods to prevent joint damage without introducing major side effects. Another common term for corticosteroids is glucocorticoids.

Synthetically produced cortisone is similar to cortisol in its activity as a corticosteroid. But prednisone is about five times more powerful than cortisone: 25 to 35 mg of cortisone are roughly equivalent to 5 to 7 mg of prednisone. Prednisone also comes in an injectable form called *Depo-Medrol* and *Solu-Medrol*. The most powerful corticosteroid is dexamethasone, which is about 10 times more powerful than cortisone: 25 mg of cortisone is equivalent to 2.5 mg of dexamethasone.

Serious side effects may occur when people take high doses of glucocorticoids over long periods. These include weight gain, a swollen or "moon face," increased susceptibility to infection, diabetes, high blood pressure, cataracts, avascular necrosis of the hip and other bones, and osteoporosis (thinning of bones). People who take high doses of corticosteroids over long periods have the same serious symptoms as those with a naturally occurring condition called *Cushing's syndrome* or *hyperadrenocorticism,* in which too much cortisol is made due to a dysregulation in the adrenal gland or due to a hormone-producing tumor.

High-Dose vs. Low-Dose Corticosteroids

One of the functions of corticosteroids is to shut down the inflammatory response after it is no longer needed to protect the body from infections or other conditions that may jump start the immune system (see Chapter 2).

Your doctor may prescribe corticosteroids to treat a variety of inflammatory conditions ranging from an acute insect bite or poison ivy to serious rheumatic diseases like rheumatoid arthritis or systemic lupus. For conditions such as asthma attacks, high doses such as 20 to 60 mg of prednisone are given, often in a "dose-pack." In this form, the amount of the drug is tapered over the course of a week to treat subacute (neither chronic nor acute) inflammatory conditions. Of course, people generally recover from these conditions, but the corticosteroids may hasten recovery, make recovery more likely, or even be life-saving. Regardless, the action of the drugs is needed for only a few days.

In a chronic condition such as rheumatoid arthritis, higher doses of corticosteroids are used over longer periods, and the situation becomes more complex. One reason is that the trigger of the inflammation continues rather than disappears. If the corticosteroid dose or dose pack is tapered rapidly and discontinued, symptoms tend to return. There may even be a strong "rebound" effect, in which symptoms actually increase. Occasionally, some physicians use high doses of pills or injections that are rapidly tapered to more normal levels to control acute flares. But over long periods, physicians try to maintain dosage at less than 5 mg of prednisone per day.

Most people with rheumatoid arthritis appear to respond to low doses of corticosteroid (such as 5 mg of prednisone or less) similar to those made naturally in the adrenal gland. The side effects of long-term, low-dose corticosteroid use are much less serious than those seen with high doses. Side effects may still be seen – thinning of the skin, bruising easily, and slower wound healing, for example – but most major consequences, such as diabetes, hypertension and weight gain, are only slightly or no more common than in the general population of people with chronic diseases.

Many rheumatoid arthritis specialists suggest that the capacity of low-dose corticosteroids to help people function from day to day, relieve pain and slow long-term joint damage makes their use worthwhile.

History of Use of Corticosteroids in Rheumatoid Arthritis

Cortisone was first produced in a laboratory in 1948. That cortisone could lead to major benefit in people with rheumatoid arthritis and other inflammatory conditions was immediately apparent. The improvement seen overnight in many people seemed almost a miracle. Popular magazine articles highlighted the dramatic effects of cortisone, and many believed a cure for rheumatoid arthritis had finally arrived.

The period of great hope lasted only a few years. By the early 1950s, doctors recognized that high doses of corticosteroids over periods longer than a few weeks or months were associated with severe side effects. The consequences often appeared to be as bad as, or even worse than, the disease itself. The medical community concluded that it would be undesirable to use any corticosteroids to treat rheumatoid arthritis. From the 1960s to the 1980s, medical texts recommended that these drugs be used only as a last resort if a person could not function at all or developed a severe consequence such as vasculitis, or inflamed blood vessels.

The medical community redefined its attitude on corticosteroids in the 1980s, when it recognized that low doses could be used over long periods with fewer side effects than those seen with high doses. The idea was not to use high-dose corticosteroids at all, but to prescribe them in low doses over long, even indefinite, periods. Researchers found that people could safely take prednisone in doses of 3 to 7.5 mg per day or less, which would yield most of the benefits of high doses with very few of the side effects. By 1992, 75 percent of people with rheumatoid arthritis under the care of rheumatologists in the United States were taking corticosteroids, mostly over long periods and in low doses.

Of course everyone is different. A few people experience psychological distress when they take any dose of corticosteroids beyond what is naturally made in the body and can't take prednisone at all. However, in some people, doses as low as 1 mg per day can be beneficial.

Discontinuing Corticosteoids – Some Precautions

Long-term use of corticosteroids in rheumatoid arthritis signals the body's adrenal glands to stop manufacturing cortisol. If someone experiences an unusual stress such as an accident, major illness or surgery, the body can't produce the boost of corticosteroids that it needs. Then it becomes necessary to give extra amounts of the drug. Likewise, a person who has taken high doses for more than a few weeks cannot abruptly stop taking them. A person may experience confusion and

even collapse from not having enough corticosteroids if they are stopped suddenly. So you must taper the dose while the adrenal glands, which make corticosteroids in the body, build up their capacity to produce normal amounts of cortisol again. This process generally takes about a month or two.

Corticosteroids by Injection

In addition to different types of corticosteroid pills, these drugs may be given by injection in several ways. Four are discussed here.

- **An intramuscular injection.** A simple injection in a muscle (known as an *intramuscular injection)* of a corticosteroid may be given to quiet a generalized flare of rheumatoid arthritis. Two compounds often used for these injections are triamcinolone (*Kenalog*) and methylprednisolone (*Depo-Medrol*). Some people receive intramuscular injections every two months rather than taking oral corticosteroids. This type of injection often results in substantial benefit, lasting from one to eight weeks. Any doctor or trained nurse can give an intramuscular injection.
- **Injection into a joint.** If a single joint is swollen out of proportion to other joints, it may be beneficial for a doctor to inject that joint directly with corticosteroid, usually

after removing as much fluid as possible (a process called *aspiration*). Joints commonly injected include the knees, ankles, shoulders, elbows, wrists and knuckles. This type of injection may be very effective for inflammation in a specific joint. The injection delivers a much higher concentration of the drug directly into the joint, and does not expose you to the potential side effects of generalized corticosteroids. Administration of an injection into a joint requires special training or experience.

- **Injection of corticosteroids in soft tissues.** Injections may be helpful for conditions such as tendinitis or bursitis (see Chapter 5) in which the site of inflammation involves the soft tissue near a joint, rather than the joint directly. For example, the drugs may be injected in the tissue around the wrist to relieve carpal tunnel syndrome, a condition which causes numbness and tingling in the fingers. A local corticosteroid injection may also be given at the base of a finger to relieve a "trigger finger" (a condition in which a finger opens suddenly with a trigger action). Corticosteroid may also be injected into tender points in people who have fibromyalgia along with rheumatoid arthritis (see Chapter 5).

- **Intravenous injection.** Intravenous corticosteroid injections, sometimes in very high doses, are known as "pulses" (or "pulse therapy"). Pulses may be given in doses up to 1,000 mg, sometimes on three consecutive days. The treatment is effective but results are temporary, and many doctors think that low-dose, long-term corticosteroids are just as helpful to people with rheumatoid arthritis. Since the introduction of many other effective treatments, the use of corticosteroid pulses has declined considerably. However, this treatment may still be effective in certain situations.

Corticosteroids as the Only Drug Treatment

Corticosteroids may leave you feeling so well that it may seem you don't need further medication. However, these drugs are rarely the only treatment for most people with rheumatoid arthritis. In general, an additional drug – usually a disease-modifying antirheumatic drug (DMARD) such as methotrexate, sulfasalazine, hydroxychloroquine or others – is needed.

What Should You Worry About When Taking Prednisone?

The side effects listed for prednisone mostly are associated with high doses of this drug, and include higher likelihood of a "moon face," weight gain, increased likelihood of developing hypertension, diabetes, osteoporosis and related fractures, and susceptibility to infections. Although these are not unusual in people who have taken high doses of prednisone, they are quite unusual in most people who have taken low doses, even over long periods. Many people have taken low-dose prednisone for more than 10 years and have normal bone densities. Rheumatoid arthritis itself increases the likelihood of infection and osteoporosis; the conditions may be a manifestation of RA but wrongly attributed to corticosteroid treatment.

Disease-Modifying Antirheumatic Drugs (DMARDs)

Disease-modifying antirheumatic drugs, or DMARDs, are a subclass of drugs that modify mechanisms in the body that may be causing your rheumatoid arthritis symptoms. Many of these drugs were first used to treat entirely different diseases, but doctors found that they also had effects that might be useful in treating arthritis.

One of the most widely used and important DMARDs for treating rheumatoid arthritis is methotrexate (*Rheumatrex, Trexall*). Disease-modifying antirheumatic drugs appear to have the capacity to slow joint destruction in rheumatoid arthritis. Disease-modifying antirheumatic drugs are used in addition to nonsteroidal anti-inflammatory drugs and often to prednisone.

One of the earliest DMARDs was injectable gold, which is still used effectively. Other DMARDs include leflunomide (*Arava*), azathioprine (*Imuran*), chloroquine, hydroxychloroquine (*Plaquenil*), sulfasalazine (*Azulfidine*), and oral gold (*Ridaura*). Another drug currently used to treat rheumatoid arthritis is not technically a DMARD, but an antibiotic: minocycline (*Minocin*). It's often included in this category when discussing rheumatoid arthritis treatment.

Methotrexate

Methotrexate was first used in the 1940s to treat various forms of cancer, including leukemia and breast cancer, and was one of the first successful chemotherapy drugs. The main action of methotrexate in cancer is to kill cells that grow and divide without control.

Rheumatoid arthritis is not a cancer, but in RA, cells in the joint don't act normally. Therefore, the idea of killing abnormally dividing cells makes sense. But killing cancer cells is different than killing cells in arthritis. If ninety-nine percent of the cancerous cells are killed, the surving one percent will usually continue to divide, returning the disease to its previous level. But in rheumatoid arthritis, if 80 percent of abnormal cells are killed, the patient usually improves greatly. So much lower amounts of methotrexate are needed to treat RA – often less than one tenth of the amount used to treat cancer.

Although the original reason for using methotrexate to treat rheumatoid arthritis involved killing abnormal cells, it now seems likely that methotrexate helps those withn rheumatoid arthritis primarily by fighting inflammation.

HIGH-DOSE AND LOW-DOSE METHOTREXATE

A simple example can help illustrate the difference between a small and large dose of methotrexate: It's like the difference between a glass versus a bottle of red wine. All bottles of wine have a warning that drinking the contents may be harmful to health, despite extensive evidence that one or two glasses a day of red wine are associated with living longer. However, one or two bottles a day of red wine will probably shorten your life. Similarly, small doses of methotrexate may be quite safe and beneficial, although large doses are appropriate only for people with cancer in certain situations.

High doses of methotrexate can come with many, severe side effects, including

hair loss, mouth sores, decreased liver function and changes in blood counts. The side effects can be dangerous and leave a person more vulnerable to infection. Low doses, however, infrequently cause changes in blood counts and liver function, although some hair loss can occur. Overall, low-dose methotrexate appears less likely to cause side effects than most drugs used in the treatment of rheumatoid arthritis, including many NSAIDs.

ARE YOU A CANDIDATE FOR METHOTREXATE?

When methotrexate was first used to treat rheumatoid arthritis, it was reserved for people whose cases were severe and long-lasting. Doctors were concerned that because of its side effects, they could not justify its use in people who had relatively mild cases of the disease. As might be expected, many of the first people to receive methotrexate as an RA treatment already had considerable joint damage. These people improved substantially, but most of them still experienced functional disability and pain from irreparably damaged joints.

After using methotrexate for 25 years as a widespread treatment for RA, doctors now realize that low doses of the drug can control inflammation and prevent damage to joints. In addition, some of the newer

RA treatments, such as leflunomide (*Arava*) and the biologic drugs, which we'll discuss later in this chapter, may be as, or more effective than methotrexate. Over the next few years, more information will emerge about the long-term effectiveness of these new drugs, and this knowledge may reshape the face of RA treatment dramatically. In addition, newer drugs may be on the horizon that will have an even greater impact.

As with all drugs, some people cannot take methotrexate. Nonetheless, with evidence of few and manageable side effects, methotrexate is one of the most common treatments for rheumatoid arthritis. Many doctors believe all people who have rheumatoid arthritis should take some dose of methotrexate if they can tolerate it. The most feared consequences – liver damage and impaired production of blood cells – are quite unusual in low doses.

WHEN SHOULD YOU BEGIN METHOTREXATE?

Here again, recommendations are changing. Traditionally, methotrexate was saved for later in the disease course. Now, with a goal of preventing damage, the drug is used early to treat inflammation as aggressively as possible. Of course, certain people may be candidates for other treatments,

such as biologic response modifiers (discussed on page 116). In addition, newer, better, and possibly safer drugs may be on the horizon for approval (see page 126).

WHEN SHOULD METHOTREXATE BE DISCONTINUED?

Although all people prefer to discontinue drug treatment if possible, considerable evidence suggests that people who respond well to methotrexate and tolerate it should continue to take some dose indefinitely. It's difficult to say you will use any drug forever, because new and better treatments may be developed or the arthritis may remit. Medical research may find a drug or treatment that people with RA need to take for only a few weeks or months rather than indefinitely. However, until such treatments become available, long-term methotrexate treatment is one of the best ways for most people to control the inflammation of rheumatoid arthritis and prevent joint damage.

WHEN SHOULD OTHER DRUGS BE ADDED?

Another shifting area of RA treatment is the combination of drugs. In the past, if you took a DMARD such as gold injections or penicillamine that seemed to work for a while and then seemed to stop working later, the doctor would discontinue that drug and begin another DMARD. Doctors felt that severe side effects were more likely if two powerful drugs were used together.

Methotrexate has far fewer side effects than most of the other drugs used to treat rheumatoid arthritis, so many doctors now add a second DMARD or biologic response modifier if methotrexate does not control swelling and pain entirely. "Combination therapy" with methotrexate and drugs such as hydroxychloroquine (*Plaquenil*), sulfasalazine (*Azulfidine*), etanercept (*Enbrel*), leflunomide (*Arava*), infliximab (*Remicade*) and others is now quite common.

Combining drugs to treat RA is similar to the way doctors manage other chronic conditions such as high blood pressure. If one drug gives partial control, they usually add a second drug rather than switching entirely from one drug to another. Sometimes a third, fourth and or even fifth drug may be added. Similarly, control of inflammation in rheumatoid arthritis may be achieved by using as many drugs as are necessary and safe.

WHAT SHOULD YOU WORRY ABOUT WHEN TAKING METHOTREXATE?

A number of warnings are often given to patients concerning the use of methotrexate, which can often be distressing. But most of the side effects are uncommon.

- **Methotrexate can reduce the formation of normal blood cells.** A check of blood cell counts is needed every four to eight weeks. However, with low-dose methotrexate, decreases in blood counts are unusual, particularly when folic acid (readily available over the counter) is used as a supplement.

- **Methotrexate is a liver toxin.** Some doctors will suggest that you completely abstain from alcohol, although other doctors think one or two alcoholic drinks per day is reasonable. All doctors agree that heavy use of alcohol is very dangerous if you're taking methotrexate. Follow your doctor's advice. Patients using methotrexate should be given liver blood tests every four to six weeks to monitor the effect of the drug on the liver.

- **Methotrexate can cause a form of pneumonia.** We usually associate pneumonia with bacteria or some other type of infection, rather than with a chemical or drug. So this possible, serious effect of methotrexate is important to note. However, after the pneumonia is better, most people can take methotrexate again a few weeks later without any problem. Some doctors believe that an infection, as well as methotrexate, may be causing the pneumonia. Nonetheless, the pneumonia gets better when you stop taking methotrexate.

Personally Speaking STORIES FROM REAL PEOPLE

"The symptoms began six years ago. In fact, RA seemed like it blew in the window one night. I was always healthy until then. I awoke with fingers that looked like sausages, so stiff that I couldn't bend them, hot and red, sore and swollen.

"Diagnosis: RA. I was devastated when the doctor told me, and as a nurse, I knew it was serious. I was sent to a rheumatologist, and treatment began immediately. I didn't adjust to having this dreadful disease well. I was depressed, and for the first time in my life, I could not do the everyday things I had taken for granted.

POSITIVE ATTITUDE: STAY ON TOP OF RA AND BEAT IT!
– LINDA KNITTLE, DECATUR, IN

"I'm now doing my best to stay active. I can't walk because of my bad feet and ankles, so I go to a pool three times a week and water walk. That way, I'm moving all my muscles and it doesn't hurt. I try to stay positive, because I will not let this disease get the best of me. I will stay on top of it and beat it.

"I pray a cure will soon come for this disease. Something more needs to be done for people that have arthritis; it's disabling and the medicines are so expensive. I will not give up. I will fight and I will hope and pray for a cure."

• **Methotrexate can cause changes in the genetic structure of cells.** Such genetic structural change in cells theoretically makes a person vulnerable to the development of cancer. However, this is unlikely when low-dose methotrexate is used for RA treatment. Many studies have shown that increased risk of cancer in methotrexate-treated patients is minimal.

• **Methotrexate is teratogenic.** Teratogenic means that the drug, taken when a woman is pregnant, ups the risk of abnormal development in a fetus. So, women of childbearing years who are not using birth control should not use methotrexate. And men should not take if either if he and his spouse are trying to conceive.

• **Methotrexate can cause hair loss.** Hair loss can often be controlled by reducing the dose. Sometimes discontinuation of the drug is necessary.

• **Methotrexate can cause mouth sores.** Mouth sores or oral ulcers are common. Again, this problem can be reduced by lowering the dosage, giving folic acid along with the methotrexate, and/or using a mouthwash treatment.

Despite the list of side effects with methotrexate treatment, more than 60 percent of people who start methotrexate take it safely for longer than five years, and more than 40 percent take it safely for more than 10 years. Low-dose methotrexate is an important, effective treatment for rheumatoid arthritis.

Biologic Response Modifiers

In the 1990s and early 21st century, several new drugs that directly modify the immune system were introduced to great fanfare: the biologic response modifiers, a new subset of DMARDs. Early recipients of the drugs often saw dramatic results, causing in one case a temporary shortage due to demand. The new group includes etanercept (*Enbrel*), infliximab (*Remicade*), anakinra (*Kineret*), adalimumab (*Humira*), abatacept (*Orencia*) and rituximab (*Rituxan*).

Biologic response modifiers specifically inhibit chemicals (called *cytokines*) that are involved in the inflammatory response. Etanercept, infliximab and adalimumab inhibit a cytokine called tumor necrosis factor, and they are often called TNF-inhibitors. Anakinra inhibits another cytokine, interleukin-1. Abatacept blocks T cells, while rituximab targets B cells. The new compounds not only relieve hard-to-treat symptoms of RA, but they also may inhibit the structural joint damage that arthritis often causes.

As we discussed earlier in the book, no case of rheumatoid arthritis is exactly like another, and no RA patient is identical to another. So despite the excitement associated with these innovative treatments, you and your doctor will still have to work together to find the particular treatment that works for you over the long-term. In many cases, combinations of new drugs and older, more established treatments still work best.

Etanercept, anakinra and adalimumab can be self-injected by the patient using prefilled devices. Infliximab, abatacept and rituximab must be infused by a health-care professional.

BRMs are still quite expensive. Insurance companies and managed-care organizations may be resistant to their use unless the disease has not been controlled with another DMARD: A drug like etanercept may cost at least 10-times as much as most of the other medications for rheumatoid arthritis.

BRMs are a major breakthrough in the treatment of RA, excellent to try as an aggressive therapy. With BRMs, total remission may be attained, something not often possible with other drugs. As all of these treatments are new and expensive compared to non-biologic drugs, consult with your insurance company to make sure the drugs are covered under your policy, and work with your doctor to get coverage if you both feel this approach is right for you.

As these new drugs have been used by RA patients for several years, some concerns have arisen. Patients with congestive heart failure (CHF) should not take adalimumab, etanercept or infliximab. Rare reports of lupus (with symptoms such as rash, fever and pleurisy) have been linked to treatment with these three drugs as well. Symptoms resolve when medication is stopped. Rarely, a neurological disease, multiple sclerosis, has developed in patients receiving biologic response modifiers. And seizures have been reported with etanercept use.

If you are exploring the use of BRMs, let your doctor know if you have or have had any of the following conditions: active infection; recurrent infection; exposure to tuberculosis or a positive skin test for tuberculosis; or a nervous system disorder such as multiple sclerosis, seizure disorders, myelitis or optic neuritis.

Etanercept

Etanercept (*Enbrel*) was the first of the BRMs, an entirely new kind of drug specifically designed to treat rheumatoid arthritis. Etanercept blocks a major component of inflammation known as tumor necrosis factor (TNF). The factor is critical in the inflammatory response. Etanercept blocks the action of TNF to help reduce inflammation.

A new study shows that RA patients taking etanercept and methotrexate in combination are much more likely to achieve clinical remission than those taking methotrexate alone. Additional studies may reveal more about the usefulness of BRMs like etanercept.

Etanercept is given twice per week as an injection under the skin. In most cases, patients inject themselves, but you can have a relative, friend or nurse do it. Side effects are minimal: etanercept is well tolerated and doesn't interfere with blood counts. There is occasional local irritation at the site of injection.

Because etanercept may block the inflammatory response too effectively, its use may make it harder for the body to fight infection. So it's recommended that you not start etanercept if you have a severe infection, and you should not take the drug if you develop an infection.

Because etanercept and other BRMs are still so new, long-term effects are unclear. Theoretically, a person may be more susceptible to cancer after taking this drug, but no evidence for this has emerged thus far. Indeed, there were similar concerns about methotrexate 15 years ago, but they have been groundless.

Etanercept is given in 50 mg weekly doses, given by subcutaneous (beneath the skin) injection. The initial dose usually is 50 mg twice per week for three months. The drug must be refrigerated. You mix the dose by injecting liquid into the vial that contains the medicine in powder form. Do not shake; instead swirl the medication prior to injection. You may inject etanercept into the thigh, abdomen or upper arm.

Possible side effects of etanercept include redness and pain; itching; swelling and/or bruising at the injection site; and upper respiratory infection.

Infliximab

Like etanercept, infliximab (*Remicade*) is designed to block the action of tumor necrosis factor (TNF) in the body. At this time, infliximab is approved by the FDA only for use in combination with methotrexate.

A new study shows that RA patients taking infliximab in combination with methotrexate have improved bone erosion scores compared to those using methotrexate alone. This finding may mean that the drug can help prevent bone erosion. Still, more tests are needed.

Infliximab is also given as an injection but in a different way from etanercept. You will receive an intravenous infusion once every one to two months in a doctor's office, specialized clinic or hospital. Infliximab is given in doses based on body weight, and ranges from 200 mg to 400 mg per treatment for most patients. The initial dose is repeated at 2 and 6 weeks and once every 8 weeks thereafter. The drug is infused intravenously (IV) during a two–hour infusion done in a doctor's office, clinical or hospital. Patients taking infliximab should also be taking methotrexate once a week by mouth or injection.

Possible infusion reactions (occurring during or shortly after the infusion) include abdominal pain, cough, dizziness, hives, itchy rash, muscle pain, nasal congestion, nausea, runny nose, shortness of breath, tightness in the chest, unusual tiredness or weakness. With infliximab, as with other BRMs, there is a mildly increased risk of common cold or upper respiratory infections.

Anakinra

Anakinra (*Kineret*) is the only biologic response modifier available that inhibits interleukin-1, an inflammatory cytokine. Like other BRMs, anakinra eases symptoms of rheumatoid arthritis and prevents joint damage.

Anakinra is given in one daily, 100 mg dose by subcutaneous (beneath the skin) injection. It can be self-injected into the thigh, abdomen or upper arm by using a traditional, prefilled syringe or an automatic injector device (*SimpleJect*) available through the drug's manufacturer. Anakinra must be refrigerated prior to use, and the syringes should not be shaken.

Similar to other BRMs, anakinra's possible side effects include injection site reactions (usually occurring during the first 4 to 6 weeks of use), including redness; swelling; pain and bruising; runny, stuffy nose; sore throat; headache; low white blood cell or platelet count.

You should discontinue anakinra if you have a serious infection (such as pneumonia) or recurrent infections. Live vaccines should not be taken along with this drug, but having a flu vaccine or vaccine for pneumonia (*Pneumovax*) is safe.

Serious infections, such as pneumonia, occur in approximately 2 percent of people taking anakinra. The percentage is possibly higher in those with asthma. If you have an infection or history of serious infection, let your doctor know before you use anakinra.

Adalimumab

Like etanercept and anakinra, adalimumab (*Humira*) can be self-injected. Like other BRMs, adalimumab appears to work well to ease RA symptoms and prevent joint damage. A new study shows that the use of adalimumab in combination with methotrexate is promising for people with long-standing RA. Additional studies may reveal more about its effectiveness and that of other BRMs.

If adalimumab is used in combination with methotrexate, the dose is 40 mg once every two weeks by subcutaneous injection. If used without methotrexate, the dose is 40 mg once a week, also by subcutaneous injection. Adalimumab, which comes in prefilled syringes, must be refrigerated until you use it.

Similar to other BRMs, which are injected or infused, possible side effects of adalimumab include redness and pain, itching, swelling and/or bruising at the injection site. It also may carry a risk of upper respiratory infection.

Like other BRMs, you should stop taking adalimumab if you have a serious infection (such as pneumonia) or recurrent infections. Do not receive live vaccines while taking this drug, although having a flu vaccine or vaccine for pneumonia (*Pneumovax*) is safe.

If you are planning to take adalimumab, let your doctor know if you have or have had any of the following: active infection; recurrent infection; exposure to tuberculosis or positive skin test for tuberculosis; a nervous system disorder, including neurological disorders such as multiple sclerosis, seizure disorders, myelitis or optic neuritis. Patients with congestive heart failure (CHF) should not take adalimumab.

Abatacept

Abatacept (*Orencia*) is used alone or in combination with other drugs for the treatment of adult patients with moderate to severe rheumatoid arthritis who have not adequately responded to other biologics. Abatacept reduces the signs and symptoms of arthritis, slows the progression of damage to the joints, and improves the physical function of patients. Abatacept should not be combined with the TNF antagonists (e.g., etanercept, adalimumab or infliximab). Abatacept blocks the activation of T cells by attaching to the protein and blocking the production of new T cells and the production of chemicals that damage tissue.

Abatacept is infused by IV over 30 minutes in a doctor's office, clinic or hospital. The dose is based on body weight and ranges from 500 to 1,000 mg. The initial dose of abatacept is followed by a second dose two weeks later with further doses every four weeks thereafter.

Common side effects include cough, dizziness, headache, sore throat and infusion reactions. Serious infections may occur. Prior to beginning treatment, you should be tested for tuberculosis. If you also have chronic obstructive pulmonary disease (COPD) and take abatacept, you should have your respiratory status monitored by your doctor.

Rituximab

Rituximab (*Rituxan*) is the latest biologic drug to be approved for the treatment of rheumatoid arthritis. It is used in combination with methotrexate to reduce the signs and symptoms of the disease in adults with moderately-to-severely active RA who have had an inadequate response to one or more TNF antagonist therapies. Rituximab previously was approved in 1997 for the treatment of CD20-positive, B-cell, non-Hodgkin's lymphoma (NHL). Rituximab is the first RA treatment that targets and selectively depletes CD20-positive B cells, which are involved in the joint inflammation that occurs in RA.

Rituximab is given as two 1,000 mg IV infusions separated by two weeks.

Administration of the intravenous corticosteroid methylprednisolone at 100 mg or its equivalent 30 minutes prior to each infusion is recommended to reduce the incidence and severity of infusion reactions. Rituximab is given in combination with methotrexate.

In clinical trials for RA, the most common adverse events observed in patients treated with rituximab were infusion reactions and infections. Severe infusion reactions, which typically occur during the first infusion, have been reported in patients treated with rituximab, some with fatal outcomes in patients with NHL.

Other Disease-Modifying Antirheumatic Drugs (DMARDs)

While BRMs have received the lion's share of attention in the health press recently, a large number of DMARDs are now available to treat RA symptoms, either in combination with methotrexate or alone. Some of these drugs are highly effective for some people with RA, and your doctor may prescribe one. Two drugs, cyclosporine and leflunomide, are chemical compounds that modify immune function and are often very effective in controlling rheumatoid arthritis symptoms. The others in this class are more traditional treatments that are often used effectively to treat RA symptoms.

Leflunomide

Leflunomide (*Arava*) is another drug that affects the immune response directly by blocking metabolic pathways important to the immune system. Leflunomide is effective for people with rheumatoid arthritis, both as a single agent and in combination with methotrexate. The typical dose of leflunomide is 100 mg for three days (a loading dose), and then 20 mg per day thereafter.

Side effects include rashes and gastrointestinal symptoms, but most common are effects on liver function. In theory, this would make combining it with methotrexate unlikely because methotrexate can also harm the liver. Research, however, has shown that methotrexate and leflunomide can be combined safely.

Although methotrexate is the most widely used DMARD, and many people are now taking some of the newer immune-response modulating drugs, other DMARDs – cyclosporine, hydroxychloroquine, sulfasalazine, injectable gold, penicillamine and azathioprine, which may be used in combination with methotrexate or another DMARD – have a place in treatment. We will also briefly discuss cyclophosphamide, which is not, strictly-speaking, a DMARD, but is used to treat potentially life-threatening forms of rheumatoid arthritis such as rheumatoid vasculitis.

Cyclosporine

Cyclosporine (*Neoral*) was originally developed to prevent organ rejection in transplant recipients. It reduces the immune response through regulatory T cells (see Chapter 2). Cyclosporine can be effective as a single drug for people with rheumatoid arthritis, or in combination with methotrexate.

Your doctor will customize the dosage of cyclosporine for you to get the most benefit and least likelihood of side effects. He or she may increase the starting dosage if no side effects on blood pressure and kidney function appear and may decrease it if they do appear, or when control of disease is excellent.

Side effects of cyclosporine include upset stomach, nausea, loss of appetite and increased hair growth. The most severe complication of cyclosporine is its effect on the kidneys. Blood pressure, which is regulated by the kidneys, may elevate and kidney function may be compromised. So, your doctor will initially monitor your kidney function with a blood test and measurement of blood

pressure every two weeks , and every month or two thereafter. Some studies also suggest long-term use of cyclosporine may increase risk of cancer.

Hydroxychloroquine

Hydroxychloroquine (*Plaquenil*) is an antimalarial drug of great benefit to some people with rheumatoid arthritis. This discovery was originally using a related compound known as chloroquine (*Aralen*). Chloroquine was given to travelers to prevent malaria. Some travelers who took chloroquine also had rheumatoid arthritis, and reported dramatic benefit. Controlled clinical trials of antimalarial drugs have also shown substantial benefit compared to placebo (or sugar pill).

A major barrier to the use of chloroquine is vision impairment in a very small number of patients. Fortunately, this is relatively rare and can be detected and addressed early with regular eye exams.

Hydroxychloroquine is derived from chloroquine and has a much lower incidence of side effects related to the eye. In fact, the likelihood of eye toxicity is lower than the likelihood of having a car accident. Eye problems do occur, but the possibility should not be a major concern for people with rheumatoid arthritis. However, people taking hydroxychloroquine should have an eye exam every year or two.

In general, antimalarial drugs are well tolerated. Gastrointestinal distress and rash sometimes occur, as is the case with almost all drugs. However, no problems with blood tests or liver or kidney function are associated with the use of antimalarial drugs.

Sulfasalazine

Sulfasalazine (*Azulfidine*) was synthesized with a goal of treating rheumatoid arthritis. It is composed of two molecular components: A sulfa molecule also found in antibiotics, and a salicylate molecule found in aspirin. Sulfasalazine is far superior to a placebo in clinical trials.

An important barrier to the use of sulfasalazine is gastrointestinal distress. Most people with rheumatoid arthritis tolerate one to two grams per day , but many people have distress when doses are raised to two to four grams per day. Sulfasalazine is often used in combinations. In fact, the combination of methotrexate, hydroxychloroquine and sulfasalazine has been found to be substantially more effective than methotrexate alone in some people.

Injectable Gold

Gold injections were the most widely used treatment for rheumatoid arthritis from the 1950s through the 1980s, and continue to be widely used in certain centers. Gold was first used early in the 20th century because doctors believed that rheumatoid arthritis might be caused by an infection (see Chapter 2), and gold was recognized as an effective treatment for infections before antibiotics were developed. During the 1930s, a French rheumatologist named Forrestier began to use gold injections systematically. His work led to the establishment of injectable gold as the major treatment for rheumatoid arthritis from the 1940s to the 1980s.

Although the injections were associated with substantial improvement in about two-thirds of patients, side effects were common: within a few months more than one-third of patients had to stop the injections because of rash, kidney problems, blood cell abnormalities and lung problems. Perhaps as important, many people who experienced a good response over three months to a year eventually stopped responding. Within two years, only about one-quarter of people who had begun gold treatment continued it.

Injectable gold is usually given as a 10-mg test dose using *Myochrysine* or *Solganol*, two different preparations of gold, followed

123

by a 25-mg dose and then a 50-mg dose at weekly intervals. If the 50-mg dose is well tolerated, the patient is treated with 50-mg injections every week for 20 weeks. The injections are then given every two weeks, three weeks or even four weeks on an indefinite basis, as long as the treatment appears effective and well tolerated and even if additional medications appear necessary. One problem in the use of gold is that its onset of action is slow; it may take three months or longer to see an effect.

Nonetheless, even after five years, about 10 to 20 percent of people who take gold injections continue to have a good response. The combination of gold with methotrexate has been studied, particularly in Europe, where results suggest it is a valuable combination for some people.

Oral Gold

Oral gold (auranofin, *Ridaura*) was developed in the 1980s as a substitute for injectable gold. In clinical trials, it was found as effective as injectable gold, but the trials involved people with rheumatoid arthritis who had not taken other DMARDs and did not have longstanding disease. So, oral gold is still used in people with early rheumatoid arthritis, but in long-term rheumatoid arthritis it does not seem as effective as many other drugs. The

side effects are similar to injectable gold, but most people tolerate oral gold better. It is sometimes used in combination with methotrexate or other DMARDs.

Azathioprine

Azathioprine (*Imuran*) was the first immunosuppressive drug approved to use for rheumatoid arthritis. It controls the production of cells that cause inflammation. At this time, azathioprine is most often used as a supplement to methotrexate or for people who cannot tolerate methotrexate because of the side effects.

Azathioprine does not appear to be as effective as methotrexate, which hypothetically has a similar mechanism of action. Doctors monitor patients who take azathioprine every four to eight weeks for altered blood counts and effects on the liver. Azathioprine has been used in combination with methotrexate, and a few people showed significant improvement. In most people, however, there was no major additional benefit from azathioprine.

Penicillamine

Penicillamine (*Depen* or *Cuprimine*) was first used in rheumatoid arthritis because it binds rheumatoid factor, although how it does this is unclear. Penicillamine is a little like gold: it is associated with occasional dramatic responses, but only about 10 percent to 20 percent of users have satisfactory long-term responses. Most doctors use a "go low, go slow" approach, beginning with 250 mg for a few weeks, and increasing the dose by 250 mg every four to eight weeks, up to 1,500 mg per day.

Although penicillamine leads to dramatic results in a few patients, its use (like the use of gold) is limited in 30 to 50 percent of patients because of side effects. The side effects include rash, inflammation of the kidney, effects on production of blood cells, gastrointestinal distress and, in a few people, a peculiar autoimmune syndrome that resembles lupus (see Chapter 3). Penicillamine has been tried in several combinations but it is not used often.

Cyclophosphamide

Cyclophosphamide (*Cytoxan*) is another immunosuppressive drug used by some rheumatologists in the 1970s in people with severe rheumatoid arthritis. Effective in many people, it also carries a likelihood of severe side effects, including a risk of sterility, bladder complications and cancer. Cyclophosphamide is a potent cytotoxic agent that leads to profound suppression of the immune system, but it is only used now in life-threatening situations, such as a vasculitis that threatens to damage or destroy the heart or kidney.

Minocycline

Although minocycline (*Minocin*) is an antibiotic and not a DMARD, and not approved by the FDA for treating rheumatoid arthritis, it is sometimes prescribed for treatment. Side effects include dizziness, vaginal infections, nausea, headache and skin rash. People who are sensitive to tetracycline medications may not want to use minocycline.

PROSORBA Column

Another treatment for rheumatoid arthritis is protein A immunoadsorption therapy, or PROSORBA Column therapy.

To administer the therapy, patients have a needle, and then a catheter, placed in each arm. Blood is drawn from one arm and run through an *apheresis machine,* a machine that separates plasma from red blood cells. The plasma is filtered through a PROSORBA Column, a plastic cylinder that contains protein A. Protein A removes antibodies and immune complexes that promote inflammation. The plasma is joined again with the red blood cells, then infused through a catheter into the other arm. The procedure is repeated weekly for 12 weeks.

125

Side effects include chills, flu-like symptoms, nausea or vomiting during the procedure and for several hours afterward. In some cases, a rash that makes it necessary to discontinue treatment. Rheumatoid arthritis may also flare briefly afterward. In the most successful cases, the rheumatoid arthritis will subside for 12 to 18 months. The treatment is given periodically over several months.

Combination Therapy

No single drug is likely to be a "magic bullet" to alleviate the inflammation and pain associated with rheumatoid arthritis. Many different types of inflammatory chemicals and abnormalities can cause inflammation in RA, so it's reasonable to imagine that at least a few different drugs may be required to control the disease. Because each DMARD works by a different mechanism , combining them may increase your ability to control inflammation and prevent joint damage.

Studies have shown that combining certain DMARDs adds considerable benefit without any need to monitor the combination more than a single DMARD and with no higher likelihood of side effects. As always, let your doctor know about any medications you are taking for conditions other than your arthritis.

By now you no doubt recognize that no single drug is best for all people with rheumatoid arthritis. Each individual is unique, and each of the drugs work better for some than for others. Some drugs are helpful to a much larger proportion of the population , but you may find one of the other drugs best for you. And certain combinations of drugs will be better for some people than others.

Research and Development: Hope for the Future

Several promising new drugs and therapies to treat rheumatoid arthritis are in development and under study. And some of the drugs discussed in this chapter are now available by prescription.

You may hear news about pharmaceutical companies researching how to treat rheumatoid arthritis and trying to develop new drugs. The process takes time: approval by the federal government's Food and Drug Administration (FDA) for a new drug results from years of testing to make sure the drug is safe and effective.

Existing treatments, including drugs used to treat diseases and conditions unrelated to arthritis, may someday be found to have a benefit for people with RA as well.

A number of new drugs designed to treat rheumatoid arthritis are in the FDA's approval process now.

A recent study conducted at the University of Glasgow in Scotland suggested that cholesterol-lowering statin drugs, such as atorvastatin calcium (*Lipitor*), may be a beneficial treatment for RA. More study is needed to confirm this. Many other treatments are in the earliest stages of research and development at pharmaceutical laboratories around the world.

You may learn about new or potential drugs on the news, or read reports on the Internet. When you hear that a drug has just been approved by the FDA, ask your doctor or other health professional for if it is a potential treatment for you.

Drugs Used in Treating Rheumatoid Arthritis

NSAIDS: NONSTEROIDAL ANTI-INFLAMMATORY DRUGS

Note: Possible side effects for all NSAIDs, except where noted, include abdominal pain; dizziness; drowsiness; fluid retention; gastric ulcers and bleeding; increased susceptibility to bruising or bleeding from cuts; heartburn; indigestion; lightheadedness; nausea; nightmares; rash; ringing in the ears; reduction in kidney function; increase in liver enzymes.

Ulcers or internal bleeding can occur without warning, so regular checkups are important. If you consume more than three alcoholic drinks per day, check with your doctor before using these products.

Aspirin
Brand names: *Anacin, Ascriptin, Bayer, Bufferin, Ecotrin, Excedrin Tablets, ZORprin, others*
Dosage: 2,400 to 5,400 mg per day in several doses

Choline and magnesium salicylates
Brand names: *CMT, Tricosal, Trilisate*
Dosage: 2,000 to 3,000 mg per day in two or three doses
Other possible side effects: Bloating, confusion, deafness, diarrhea

Choline salicylate
Brand name: *Arthropan*
Dosage: 3,480 mg or 20 ml per day in several doses
Other possible side effects: Bloating, confusion, deafness, diarrhea

Diclofenac potassium
Brand name: *Cataflam*
Dosage: 100 to 200 mg per day in two or four doses

Diclofenac sodium
Brand name: *Voltaren, Voltaren XR*
Dosage: 100 to 200 mg per day in two or four doses (Voltaren); 100 mg in single daily dose (*Voltaren XR*)

Diflunisal
Brand name: *Dolobid*
Dosage: 500 to 1,500 mg per day in two doses

Etodolac
Brand names: *Lodine, Lodine XL*
Dosage: 600 to 1,200 mg per day in two or four doses (Lodine); 400 to 1,000 mg per day in a single dose for (*Lodine XL*)

Fenoprofen calcium
Brand name: *Nalfon*
Dosage: 900 to 2,400 per day in three or four doses; never more than 3,200 mg per day

Flurbiprofen
Brand name: *Ansaid*
Dosage: 200 to 300 mg per day in two or four doses

Ibuprofen
Brand names: *Advil, Motrin, Motrin IB, Mediprin, Nuprin*
Dosage: 1,200 to 3,200 mg per day in three or four doses for prescription-strength Motrin; 200 to 400 mg every four to six hours as needed, not exceeding 1,200 mg per day, for over-the-counter brands

Indomethacin
Brand name: *Indocin, Indocin SR*
Dosage: 50 to 200 mg per day in two to four doses for Indocin; 75 mg per day in one dose, or 150 mg per day in two doses for Indocin SR.
Other possible side effects: Depression, headache, "spacey" feeling

Ketoprofen
Brand names: *Actron, Orudis, Orudis-KT, Oruvail*
Dosage: 200 to 225 mg per day in three or four doses for *Orudis*; 150 or 200 mg per day in a single dose for *Oruvail*; 12.5 mg every four to six hours as needed for *Actron* and *Orudis-KT*

Magnesium salicylate
Brand names: *Magan, Doan's Pills, Mobidin, Arthritab*
Dosage: 2,600 to 4,800 mg per day in three to six doses
Other possible side effects: Bloating, confusion, deafness, diarrhea

Meclofenamate sodium
Brand name: *Meclomen*
Dosage: 200 to 400 mg per day in four doses

Mefenamic acid
Brand name: *Ponstel*
Dosage: 250 mg every six hours as needed, for up to seven days

Meloxicam
Brand name: *Mobic*
Dosage: 7.5 to 15 mg per day in a single dose

Drugs Used in Treating Rheumatoid Arthritis (cont.)

Nabumetone
Brand name: *Relafen*
Dosage: 1,000 mg per day in one or two doses, or 2,000 mg per day in two doses

Naproxen
Brand names: *Naprosyn, Naprelan*
Dosage: 500 to 1,500 mg per day in two doses for *Naprosyn*; 750 or 1,000 mg per day in a single dose for *Naprelan*

Naproxen sodium
Brand names: *Anaprox, Aleve*
Dosage: 550 to 1,650 mg per day in two doses for *Anaprox*; 220 mg every eight to 12 hours as needed for *Aleve*

Oxaprozin
Brand name: *Daypro*
Dosage: 1,200 mg or 1,800 mg per day in a single dose

Piroxicam
Brand name: *Feldene*
Dosage: 20 mg per day in one or two doses

Salsalate
Brand names: *Disalcid, Mono-gesic, Salflex, Salsitab, Arnigesic, Anaflex 750, Marthritic*
Dosage: 1,000 to 3,000 mg per day in two or three doses
Other possible side effects: Bloating, confusion, deafness, diarrhea

Sodium salicylate
Brand name: *None, generic only*
Dosage: 3,600 to 5,400 mg per day in several doses
Other possible side effects: Bloating, confusion, deafness, diarrhea

Sulindac
Brand name: *Clinoril*
Dosage: 300 to 400 mg per day in two doses

Tolmetin sodium
Brand name: *Tolectin*
Dosage: 1,200 mg to 1,800 mg per day in three doses

COX-2 INHIBITORS

Celecoxib
Brand name: *Celebrex*
Dosage: 200 mg per day in one or two doses or 400 mg per day in two doses
Possible side effects: Same as other NSAIDS, except less likely to cause gastric ulcers and susceptibility to bruising and bleeding. Also potential risk of heart attack, stroke, blood clots or some skin reactions.

ANALGESICS

Except for than acetaminophen, these pain-relieving drugs have the potential for dependence if used for long periods.

Acetaminophen
Brand names: *Anacin (aspirin-free), Excedrin caplets, Panadol, Tylenol*
Dosage: 325 to 1,000 mg every four to six hours as needed; no more than 4,000 mg per day
Possible side effects: When taken as prescribed, acetaminophen is not usually associated with side effects

Acetaminophen with codeine
Brand names: *Fioricet, Phenaphen with codeine, Tylenol with codeine #3*
Dosage: 15 to 60 mg every four hours as needed
Possible side effects: Constipation, dizziness or lightheadedness, drowsiness, nausea, unusual tiredness or weakness, vomiting

Propoxyphene hydrochloride
Brand names: *Darvon, PC-Cap, Wygesic*
Dosage: 65 mg every four hours as needed; no more than 390 mg per day
Possible side effects: Dizziness or lightheadedness, drowsiness, nausea and vomiting

Tramadol
Brand name: *Ultram*
Dosage: 50 to 100 mg every four to six hours as needed
Possible side effects: Dizziness, nausea, constipation, headache, sleepiness

Tramadol with acetaminophen
Brand name: *Ultracet*
Dosage: 75 mg every four to six hours as needed for up to five days; no more than 300 mg per day
Possible side effects: Constipation, diarrhea, dizziness, drowsiness, increased sweating, loss of appetite, nausea

Drugs Used in Treating Rheumatoid Arthritis (cont.)

CORTICOSTEROIDS

Note: Side effects may be minimal when corticosteroids are taken short-term or at very low doses. The following side effects are possible for the following corticosteroids, but are more common with high doses and long-term use: Cushing's syndrome (weight gain, moon-face, thin skin, muscle weakness, brittle bones), cataracts, hypertension, increased appetite, elevated blood sugar, indigestion, insomnia, mood changes, nervousness or restlessness.

Dosage varies greatly based on disease severity. Take the amount prescribed by your doctor.

Cortisone
Brand names: *Cortone*
Dosage: 5 to 150 mg per day in a single dose

Dexamethasone
Brand names: *Decadron, Hexadrol*
Dosage: 0.5 to 9 mg per day in a single dose

Hydrocortisone
Brand names: *Cortef, Hydrocortone*
Dosage: 20 to 240 mg per day in a single dose or divided into several doses

Methylprednisolone
Brand name: *Medrol*
Dosage: 4 to 160 mg per day in a single dose or divided into several doses

Prednisolone
Brand name: *Prelone*
Dosage: 5 to 200 mg per day in a single dose or divided into several doses

Prednisolone sodium phosphate (liquid only)
Brand name: *Pediapred*
Dosage: 5 to 60 ml per day in one to three doses

Prednisone
Brand names: *Deltasone, Orasone, Prednicen-M, Sterapred*
Dosage: 1 to 60 mg per day in a single dose or divided into several doses

Triamcinolone
Brand name: *Aristocort*
Dosage: 4 to 60 mg per day in a single dose or divided into several doses

BIOLOGIC RESPONSE MODIFIERS

Abatacept
Brand name: *Orencia*
Dosage: 500 to 1,000 mg per treatment, based on body weight
Possible side effects: cough; dizziness; headache; infusion reactions, including change in blood pressure, facial swelling, hives, trouble breathing; serious infections; sore throat

Adalimumab
Brand name: *Humira*
Dosage: 40 mg injected beneath the skin every other week in combination with methotrexate; 40 mg once a week when used alone.
Possible side effects: Redness and pain; itching; swelling and/or bruising at the injection site; upper respiratory infection

Anakinra
Brand name: *Kineret*
Dosage: Injected beneath the skin in daily 100-mg doses.
Possible side effects: Skin reactions, including pain, swelling and redness and the injection site

Etanercept
Brand name: *Enbrel*
Dosage: Injected beneath the skin in 25 mg doses twice per week, or 50 mg given in two daily 25 mg doses (separate sites)
Possible side effects: Redness and/or itching; pain or swelling at the injection site

Infliximab
Brand name: *Remicade*
Dosage: Determined by body weight. Drug is infused intravenously in a two-hour outpatient procedure every one to two months. Only approved for use in combination with methotrexate.
Possible side effects: Upper respiratory infection, headache, nausea, coughing

Rituximab
Brand name: *Rituxan*
Dosage: Two 1,000 mg doses infused intravenously separated by two weeks. Only approved for use in combination with methotrexate.
Possible side effects: Infusion reactions, infection

Drugs Used in Treating Rheumatoid Arthritis (cont.)

DMARDs – DISEASE-MODIFYING ANTIRHEUMATIC DRUGS – AND OTHERS

Note: Minocycline, an antibiotic, is included here, since it is effective in treating rheumatoid arthritis. Many DMARDs are used in combination to increase effectiveness and decrease side effects. Comprehensive explanations of cautions are in this chapter.

Auranofin (oral gold)
Brand name: *Ridaura*
Dosage: 6 to 9 mg per day in one or two doses
Possible side effects: Abdominal or stomach cramps or pain; bloated feeling; decrease in or loss of appetite; diarrhea or loose stools; gas or indigestion; mouth sores; nausea or vomiting; skin rash or itching

Azathioprine
Brand name: *Imuran*
Dosage: 50 to 150 mg per day in one to three doses, based on body weight
Possible side effects: Cough, fever and chills; loss of appetite; nausea or vomiting; skin rash; unusual bleeding or bruising; unusual tiredness or weakness

Cyclophosphamide
Brand name: *Cytoxan*
Dosage: 50 to 150 mg per day in a single dose; may also be given intravenously
Possible side effects: Blood in urine or burning on urination; confusion or agitation; cough; dizziness; fever and chills; infertility in men and women; loss of appetite; missed menstrual periods; nausea or vomiting; unusual bleeding or bruising; unusual tiredness or weakness

Cyclosporine
Brand names: *Sandimmune, Neoral*
Dosage: 100 to 400 mg per day in two doses; dose is based on body weight
Possible side effects: Tender or enlarged gums; high blood pressure; increase in hair growth; kidney problems; loss of appetite, tremors

Injectable gold
Brand names: *Gold sodium thiolomate: Myochrysine; Aurothioglucose: Solganol*
Dosage: 10 mg in a single dose the first week, 25 mg the following week, then 25 to 50 mg per week thereafter. Frequency may be reduced after several months.
Possible side effects: Irritation or soreness on the tongue; metallic taste; skin rash or itching; soreness; swelling or bleeding of gums; unusual bleeding or bruising

Hydroxychloroquine sulfate
Brand name: *Plaquenil*
Dosage: 200 to 600 mg per day in one or two doses
Possible side effects: Black spots in visual field, diarrhea, loss of appetite, nausea, rash

Leflunomide
Brand name: *Arava*
Dosage: 10 to 20 mg per day in a single dose
Possible side effects: Diarrhea, skin rash, liver toxicity, hair loss

Methotrexate
Brand name: *Rheumatrex, Trexall*
Dosage: 7.5 to 20 mg per week in a single dose taken orally; may also be given by injection
Possible side effects: Cough; diarrhea; hair loss; loss of appetite; unusual bleeding or bruising; liver toxicity; lung toxicity

Minocycline
Brand name: *Minocin*
Dosage: 200 mg per day in two doses
Possible side effects: Dizziness, vaginal infections, nausea, headache, skin rash

Penicillamine
Brand names: *Cuprimine, Depen*
Dosage: 125 to 250 mg per day in a single dose to start, increased to not more than 1,500 mg per day in three doses
Possible side effects: Diarrhea, joint pain, lessening or loss of sense of taste, loss of appetite, fever, hives or itching, mouth sores, nausea or vomiting, skin rash, stomach pain, swollen glands, unusual bleeding or bruising, weakness

Sulfasalazine
Brand name: *Azulfidine, Azulfidine EN–Tabs*
Dosage: 500 to 3,000 mg per day in two to four doses
Possible side effects: Stomach upset, diarrhea, dizziness, headache, light sensitivity, itching, appetite loss, liver abnormalities, lowered blood count, rash, nausea or vomiting

For more arthritis drug information, The Arthritis Foundation publishes the book *Essential Guide to Arthritis Medications*, available for purchase by calling 800-283-7800, or online at www.arthritis.org.

Chapter 12

Surgical Options:
Opening New Doors

For many people with rheumatoid arthritis, surgery is an important treatment option. In addition to other parts of their long-term treatment, such as drugs, exercise, physical and occupational therapy, and joint protection, surgery can improve function and reduce pain in many joints affected by the disease.

Surgical procedures for people with arthritis are becoming more effective and sophisticated. New technology and advances in surgical techniques as well as the composition of joint replacement parts are making surgery a more important area of arthritis treatment than ever before. The development of surgical options for arthritis over the last 35 years is one of the major breakthroughs in helping people remain active and continue to enjoy life after their diagnosis.

People with RA can face surgery at various points in the course of their disease. For example, in the early stages of the disease, a synovectomy (the surgical removal of the synovium, or lining of the joint) may be performed when one or two joints are affected by inflammation more than other joints. In later stages, an arthrodesis or fusion of a joint may greatly relieve pain. If severe damage of a joint (most commonly a hip or knee) has occurred, a total joint replacement or arthroplasty may dramatically relieve pain and improve a person's ability to function. As doctors apply the aggressive, early treatment philosophy and prescribe new drugs that may prevent joint damage, some surgical procedures may become less prevalent — even obscure. But for now, surgery remains a viable, important treatment option.

In this chapter, we discuss the main procedures used to treat RA and talk about what to expect from surgery.

Remember: each person is different. No two people will have the same outcome from or experience of surgery and rehabilitation. You'll learn here what you can do before and after the operation to increase the chances of surgical success. We will also provide additional resources for you to explore as you consider joint surgery.

Common Surgical Procedures

In the coming sections, we'll discuss the most important surgical procedures for treating rheumatoid arthritis. Your rheumatologist will refer you to an orthopaedic surgeon to perform your surgery. These physicians specialize in surgical procedures involving bone, joints, and soft tissues surrounding bones and joints. Your orthopaedic surgeon will guide you through preparation, the procedure itself, initial recovery, and your long-term rehabilitation. You will likely work with a physical therapist (PT) during your rehabilitation.

Here are the most common surgical procedures for rheumatoid arthritis treatment. For more in-depth exploration of joint surgery, read *All You Need to Know About Joint Surgery* published by the Arthritis Foundation. See the back of this book for more information.

Synovectomy

The synovium is the protective lining of the joint. When one or two joints, such as a wrist or knee, stands out as much more severely involved than other joints, your doctor may suggest a synovectomy. This procedure is designed to remove diseased synovium and reduce the amount of inflammatory tissue, relieving swelling and pain. Synovectomy may slow or prevent damage to the joint, but the synovium may grow back after several years, causing the problem to recur.

Synovectomies are usually performed in the wrist, elbow or knee, and may be combined with resection (see page 140). If inflammation has caused tendons to rupture, then your surgeon may repair and reconstruct those tendons simultaneously to improve function. Tendon rupture is unusual except in people with rheumatoid arthritis or cases of injury.

Arthroscopic Surgery

An arthroscope is an instrument that consists of a very thin tube with a light at the end that a surgeon inserts into the joint through a small incision. Arthroscopic surgery has become more and more common over the last 20 years because it involves smaller incisions than traditional surgery, leading to a quicker recovery in most people. In addition, certain types of repairs can be done more easily with an arthroscope. A recent study questioned the value of some minor arthroscopic procedures, but most doctors feel the procedures can be useful in arthritis cases.

Arthroscopy allows the surgeon to view the inside of a joint. The arthroscope is connected to a closed-circuit television, allowing the doctor to see inside the joint and estimate the extent of damage. The doctor then has many options, including taking samples of tissue for laboratory analysis, removing pieces of loose cartilage or other tissue that can cause pain, repairing a tear in the cartilage, smoothing a rough joint surface, or performing a synovectomy, which removes diseased synovial tissue (described earlier).

Arthroscopic surgery can hypothetically be performed in any joint, but most commonly in the knee and shoulder.

Arthroplasty, or Joint Replacement Surgery

Of all the types of surgery available for people with arthritis, you've most likely heard about this one. That's because joint replacement surgery is one of the biggest success stories in the treatment of chronic joint diseases like rheumatoid arthritis. Joint replacement surgery – or arthroplasty – is the surgical reconstruction or replacement of a joint.

Joint replacement is available for many different joints but most commonly performed on the hip or knee. Joint replacement surgery has been extremely successful in enabling people, otherwise destined for a wheelchair, to continue mobility and independence. Joint replacement is recommended most often for people older than age 50, but people whose rheumatoid arthritis developed in childhood or at an early age may require joint reconstruction sooner.

The procedure itself involves removing the damaged joint, resurfacing and relining the ends of bones where cartilage has worn away, and replacing the joint with one of several types of man-made components made of metal, ceramic or plastic parts.

Two categories of replacement joints are used: cemented or cementless. Cemented joints are secured during surgery with a special cementing material called *methylmethacrylate*. Cementless joints usually have a porous surface that is fitted next to the bone. Over time, the bone will grow into the joint and hold it in place. In general, cementless replacements are thought to last longer than cemented joints. In addition, they usually lead to better bone remodeling (the regrowth of bone around the prosthetic

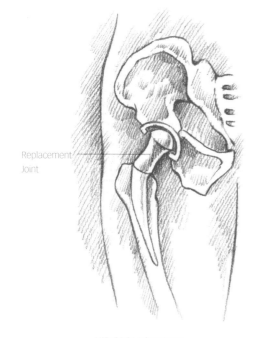

Replacement
Joint

HIP REPLACEMENT

years or more. In fact, in many people a replacement joint may last indefinitely. If the joint replacement breaks down, revision arthroplasty is often successful, and further replacement unnecessary.

New surgical procedures are making some forms of joint replacement surgery less invasive, requiring smaller incisions and shorter, easier recovery. Computer-assisted arthroplasty is on the rise, making the procedures more precise. The innovation and research in this field is plentiful, so in the years to come, joint replacement surgery will become a much easier enterprise for a person with arthritis.

Resection

Resection is a procedure that involves removing all or part of a bone. Most commonly used years ago to relieve pain and improve function in the hands and wrists in early rheumatoid arthritis, and to protect the tendons from damage, it was often combined with synovectomy. Resection of damaged joints in the feet is still commonly performed to remove bunions in the large toe or hammer toes in the other toes. Resection can make walking less painful by removing parts of a bone that causes pressure.

Resection is sometimes used in conjunction with joint replacement – a procedure known as *resection arthroplasty*.

joint) and easier revision, or replacement, if necessary. However, uncemented joint replacements usually require a longer period on crutches or using a cane after surgery. So your decision about using cemented or cementless replacement also depends on your lifestyle or occupation.

Unfortunately, joint replacements may not last forever. The cement may loosen, or one of the components may break. In the early days of joint replacement surgery, about 30 years ago, the replaced joint lasted only five to 10 years. But improvements in both artificial joints and surgical techniques have expanded that 15

However, this type of surgery is rarely used as a primary procedure; surgeons have developed more successful types of joint replacement surgery. Resection procedures are used commonly only on the feet.

Arthrodesis (Fusion)

Arthrodesis is a surgical procedure that fuses two bones. Although arthrodesis limits movement, it is usually done to relieve pain and to increase stability in the ankles, wrists, fingers and toes. It may also be performed in the spine, fusing two or more vertebrae to stabilize the spine and eliminate pain. In rare situations when joint replacement surgery is unsuccessful or results in an infection, or if surrounding structures are destroyed, arthrodesis of the hip or knee can provide another surgical option.

In arthrodesis, the bones forming a joint are joined together, often using bones from the patient's pelvis – or sometimes metallic or plastic hardware – to hold the bones together until they begin to grow and fuse. The resulting fused joint will lose flexibility, but will be less painful, more stable and often more capable of function such as bearing weight.

Osteotomy

The term *osteotomy* means "to cut bone." The procedure has often been used when

joints are malaligned, or do not line up correctly, as a result of damage to supporting structures and bone. Osteotomy increases stability by redistributing weight on the joint. Most surgeons perform osteotomy in the hip or knee to shift the load of bearing weight from areas where the cartilage is damaged to areas that still have cartilage to cushion the load. Surgeons cut the bones whose ends do not line up and repositioning them to improve alignment.

Because of better control of inflammation, leading to fewer alignment problems, and improvements in joint replacement surgery, osteotomies are much less common. In general, osteotomies are most successful in young active people who have a good range of motion in the joint, good muscle function and some cartilage around the joint.

What You Can Expect From Surgery

In most cases, surgery for people with rheumatoid arthritis is an elective procedure, performed by choice and not because of medical urgency or a life-threatening situation (such as an inflamed appendix). Nevertheless, this medically important procedure may dramatically relieve pain and restore lost function and independence.

Deciding on Surgery

Suppose your doctor has suggested that you may benefit from undergoing one of the surgical procedures discussed above. Most likely, you will have time to consider your decision and discuss options with your doctor and the surgeon. Surgery may seem scary, but it is often the best treatment to help you lead a normal life.

Because you may have weeks to wait between the time you schedule an elective joint replacement procedure and the surgery itself, you will also have time to find out more about the surgery ahead of time – including risks, details about how the procedure is done, the expected recovery time and the ways you can participate. As with all treatments, consider the risks as well as the benefits. Risks associated with joint surgery include:

- **Anesthesia.** Certain risks are associated with the use of general anesthesia, especially if you have heart disease or a chronic lung condition. General anesthesia slows heartbeat and breathing rates so those are monitored during surgery. And it causes your blood vessels to widen, which can cause heavier blood loss during the surgery. Be sure to discuss these and other risks with your surgeon and anesthesiologist before the surgery.

- **Blood clots.** These can develop following surgery, particularly if the surgery is in your lower extremities. Blood clots are less common than they once were due to improvements in postoperative care.
- **Infection.** An infection can be introduced into the joint, jeopardizing the replacement's success. In rare instances, the infection may spread to other parts of your body via the bloodstream.
- **Weight.** The stress of excess weight on a weight-bearing joint can slow recovery from surgery and cause problems during the surgery itself, making the procedure more difficult and increasing the risk of complications such as infection in the incision, lungs and other organs.

In addition to these general risks, a person with rheumatoid arthritis may encounter some particular problems with surgery. The drug program used to treat rheumatoid arthritis often must be adjusted prior to surgery. For instance, you may be asked to stop taking NSAIDs and methotrexate for the week prior to surgery, or to lower the dose. Such changes be carefully planned prior to surgery so that you can avoid a sudden flare of disease. And in some cases, people may need multiple surgeries, for instance, surgery in the foot

THAT MINTY-FRESH FEELING
– BARBARA REYNOLDS, HOLLAND PATENT, NY

"We were visiting our daughter and her family in Michigan in our RV, and our grand-children, ages 4 and 7, wanted to stay overnight with Nana and Grampa. The two children slept with me, and Grampa slept up front. During the night, my knee and hip began to hurt. I reached for my rub in the dark, so I wouldn't wake anyone. I got my tube and rubbed from knee to my hip. Boy, did I smell good! But I still hurt. I turned on the light and realized that I had reached for the toothpaste. My granddaughter will not let me forget my new arthritis rub!"

and ankle before a total knee replacement, so that rehabilitation will go well.

Before Surgery

Once you have decided to go ahead with surgery, you will need to make plans for the procedure. Your doctor's office will handle administrative details, such as getting preapprovals for surgery. Many orthopaedic surgeons conduct educational programs about surgery, including classes, videos or individualized instruction that can be very helpful.

The following page provides a list of questions to think about during such education programs and to discuss with your doctor or other health professionals as you prepare for surgery. Answers to the questions can help you decide about surgery

and know what to expect before, during and after the procedure.

After Surgery

As with any component of your arthritis management plan, surgery – or rather, recovery from surgery – requires your participation for the best results. The procedure is merely the first step in a longer process of rehabilitating the joint. The end result is worth the effort. Surgeries for arthritis relieve pain and improve joint function.

Some are more complicated than others with longer recoveries. For example, rehabilitation after knee replacement requires more effort than rehabilitation after hip replacement – and recovery takes longer. In general, your surgeon and physical therapist will advise you to begin moving your affected joint as soon as possible, sometimes even before your sutures heal. Movement should be gentle at first, increasing as appropriate.

Within a few weeks, you should be able to return to most of your daily activities. Following joint replacement surgery, recovery may take longer, and your doctor may ask you not to do certain activities for several months. Every person recovers differently; but returning to full-time activities is usually possible within three months.

For any surgery to be successful, you must be serious and committed about your rehabilitation. Rehabilitation of a surgically repaired joint can be tedious, but it is also critical. A physical or occupational therapist usually guides your rehabilitation. In some cases, a patient begins therapy in a hospital or postoperative rehabilitation facility, but many attend therapy sessions in an office setting. But only a small part of rehabilitation occurs in a hospital, doctor's or therapist's office. You'll do most of the exercise routine at home – and part of your job will be to keep yourself motivated and to do your exercises regularly. The payoff is proportional to the amount of work you do.

Checklist: Questions to Ask Before Surgery

1. Do I understand the procedure? Are there written materials, classes or videos of the surgery that I can review ?

2. Can I talk with someone who has experienced the procedure with this orthopaedic surgeon?

3. Will I be an inpatient (a patient requiring an overnight stay) or outpatient (a patient who goes home the same day as the surgery)? If I will be an inpatient, how long might I be hospitalized?

4. Are there minimally invasive procedures available for the type of surgery I need?

5. What are the risks involved ? How likely are they to occur? Do I have any special risk factors?

6. Will I need to lose weight before my surgery – or to qualify for surgery? If so, can you guide me in this effort?

7. What are the risks if I delay or choose not to have the surgery?

8. Is it likely that more surgery will be necessary? If revision surgery is needed, what will that mean? When might that occur?

9. What improvement can I expect from surgery? Is there any downside to this procedure (for example, loss of joint motion following arthrodesis)?

10. Will I need to stop taking any of my medications before surgery? How long before?

11. Can I arrange to have blood taken from me weeks before surgery so that if I need a blood transfusion because of blood loss during surgery, it can be my own blood (the safest form of transfusion)?

12. How much pain should I expect? How long will it last? How will my pain be treated in the hospital and afterward?

13. What exercise program is recommended before and after the operation?

14. When do I start physical therapy? Will I do it myself at home or at the therapist's office? Will you refer me to a physical therapist?

15. Will I need to arrange for assistance at home after the surgery? For how long?

16. Will I need any special equipment at home? Do I need to make any modifications in my home, such as installing grab bars or ramps?

17. How will my activities – driving, climbing stairs, returning to work, having sex – be limited and for how long?

18. How often will I have follow-up visits? Will my rheumatologist be involved as well?

Chapter 13

Alternative Therapies:
Treatment's Old and New Frontier

One of several messages we hope you get from this book is that answers for the complex problems caused by rheumatoid arthritis are not simple. Rheumatoid arthritis affects each person differently, making treatment decisions sometimes seem arbitrary. Standard or conventional medicine has no cures for arthritis, as it does for infections, stomach ulcers and other diseases.

Because of this, the issue of complementary and alternative therapies has always been a subtext of treatment.

Study after study has shown that people with arthritis turn to these therapies, in part because drugs do not control disease symptoms completely and because patients are dissatisfied with the present health care system. In fact, according to a 2002 survey conducted by a number of government agencies including the National Institutes of Health, 36 percent of American use some kind of unconventional, alternative or complementary therapy. When prayer for one's health is added, the percent jumps to 62 percent. A 2004 British study showed that 44 percent of RA patients surveyed used herbal and OTC treatments.

According to most definitions, an alternative therapy is any practice or substance outside the realm of conventional medicine. Complementary therapy includes practices that coexist with traditional treatment.

Alternative therapies can provide a sense of direction and control to people who have chronic health conditions. Some of the treatments, however, conflict with accepted scientific principles and natural laws. When accompanied by aggressive or misleading marketing tactics that promise a "cure" for arthritis, the therapies alarm many doctors who tended to react negatively and refuse to discuss the therapies with their patients.

With the establishment of the National Institutes of Health Office of Alternative Medicine in 1992, now known as the National Center for Complementary and Alternative Medicine (NCCAM), many alternative therapies are better understood. Many health-care providers now realize their patients are trying unconventional remedies and that discussing them – and their potential effects – with patients is better than ignoring the issue.

Discussing the dozens (perhaps hundreds) of complementary and alternative therapies in a single chapter would be impossible. Instead, we present some broad categories of unconventional therapies, offering information that can help you discuss the topic with your doctor and make informed choices. For more in-depth information about individual therapies, see the Arthritis Foundation's book, *Alternative Treatments for Arthritis: An A to Z Guide*.

Types of Complementary And Alternative Therapy

(Note to reader: Relaxation and stress reduction techniques, such as guided imagery and relaxation exercises are discussed in Chapter 18. Exercise is covered in Chapter 14. Because these complementary therapies are an important part of a comprehensive arthritis management program, we cover them more thoroughly in those chapters.)

Massage

Many health professionals consider massage an excellent way to ease pain and stiffness associated with arthritis. It can help stretch tight muscles, improve flexibility, and ease pain and stress. Massage is usually categorized as a complementary therapy; in fact, rheumatologists often recommend

Learn More About Alternative Treatments

The Arthritis Foundation's *Alternative Treatments for Arthritis: An A to Z Guide* ($13.95) offers reliable answers to your questions about 111 forms of alternative and complementary treatments for arthritis, including supplements, acupuncture, tai chi, yoga, chiropractic, meditation, magnet therapy and more. You can order the book from the Arthritis Foundation by calling 800-283-7800 or on www.arthritis.org.

massage for arthritis and related conditions. Evidence from scientific studies has shown that massage can decrease stress hormones and depression, ease muscle pain and spasms, increase the body's production of natural pain-killing endorphins, and improve sleep and immune function.

Although many different types of massage are available, most include a combination of strokes, friction and pressure to relax the muscles. Some types, such as Swedish massage, emphasize the physical by using pressing, rubbing and manipulation, working on muscles and joints to improve function. Asian techniques emphasize balancing the flow of energy in your body. Some techniques – such as reiki and therapeutic touch –focus on channeling spiritual energy, and practitioners don't physically touch you at all.

What can you expect from your massage? Your session may take place in a softly lit, warm room with quiet music, or in a typical doctor's office. Before starting, the therapist may talk to you about any special health conditions or sensitivities (such as inflamed or painful joints), and discuss your goals for the session. You'll then lie down on a padded table or a mat on the floor for the massage. You do not have to remove all of your clothes; often, the therapist will cover you with a large sheet, uncovering only the part of your body that is being massaged.

Sessions vary from 45 to 90 minutes, and cost from $50 to $100 per hour (although prices vary by location and expertise of the therapist). During that time, the therapist will periodically ask how you are or tell you what to do. You should speak up any time you feel pain or discomfort, or if you have questions. After the session, most people feel relaxed but energized. Any soreness from the massage should disappear by the next day. If it does not, discuss it with your therapist before the next session.

Although massage is beneficial for many people, use caution when choosing a therapist. Therapists may not have experience working on people with rheumatoid arthritis and may not understand their physical needs. Some elements of massage such as strong finger pressure may not be appropriate for people with rheumatoid arthritis. And massage on an inflamed joint may make it feel worse. Another caveat: massage may not be covered by your insurance policy, even when your doctor recommends it.

Acupuncture/Acupressure

Long a cornerstone of Chinese medicine, acupuncture has entered the Western world as a treatment of many chronic conditions, including rheumatoid arthritis. In acupuncture, disposable stainless steel needles stimulate specific points located in energy pathways, or *meridians* throughout the body. The pathways have no counterpart in conventional medicine and anatomy.

More than 15 million Americans have used acupuncture, primarily for pain relief. Studies suggest that acupuncture may lessen pain by causing the body to release endorphins (naturally produced chemicals that block pain messages and prevent them from reaching the brain). Acupuncture may also have anti-inflammatory effects, but further research is needed to document this.

Acupuncture sessions usually last 30 to 60 minutes (longer on your first visit) and may cost up to $75 per session. You will be asked to sit or lie on a padded table, to remove or loosen clothing, and to get comfortable before treatment starts. A traditional Chinese acupuncture practitioner may ask you many questions about your health, diet and sleep habits. For the treatment itself, the practitioner will use from two to 15 thin needles, inserted at specific points that relate to your condition in Chinese medicine. The treatment may be combined with heat or gentle electrical stimulation.

You should not feel pain, although you may experience slight discomfort when the needles are inserted. The acupuncturist will leave you resting with the needles in place for a short period (20 minutes is typical). Once the needles are removed, you will rest briefly before getting up.

Although the World Health Organization has endorsed the use of acupuncture to treat rheumatoid arthritis, many studies have failed to document the therapy's effectiveness. If you decide to try acupuncture, find a practitioner who is certified or licensed. Some health insurers will cover the treatments if they are prescribed (or performed) by a doctor. In addition, make sure that the practitioner uses only sterile, disposable needles.

The idea of having someone insert needles into your body is unappealing. Many people get some of the same benefits from acupressure, an older form of this therapy. Instead of needles, practitioners use their fingers or other tools to apply pressure to the same points used in acupuncture.

Special Diets or Dietary Changes

The myth of the miracle arthritis diet is one of the oldest touted alternative therapies. However, scientific studies have never shown that any specific diet alone can control any form of arthritis, with the exception of gout. However, diet undeniably affects our health, and what we eat plays a role in many disorders. In addition, several research studies indicate that in some people with rheumatoid arthritis some foods make their symptoms better and others make their symptoms worse. No consistent patterns were identified in all patients.

Ways in which diet might affect your arthritis:

- **Food sensitivities.** A small number of people with arthritis might be sensitive to certain foods that could trigger symptoms or cause them to worsen.
- **Saturated fats.** A diet high in saturated fats or vegetable oils can increase the inflammatory response, contributing to joint and tissue inflammation.
- **Overall health.** Diet affects your health and any other diseases or conditions you may have (such as diabetes or heart disease). This, in turn, may affect how your body handles arthritis symptoms.
- **Poor nutrition.** Just having arthritis can make your diet worse. How? You may be unable to shop for and prepare nutritious food. Pain and fatigue can diminish your appetite or make food difficult to eat and chew.

Many fad diets claim to alleviate arthritis – everything from fasting to elimination diets (that is, eliminating a certain food or food group from your diet, such as dairy products). The few well-structured research studies concerning diet indicate that what seems to work for one person with rheumatoid arthritis may not work for another. So don't try any extreme dietary changes. But if you notice that eating a food makes your arthritis better or worse, don't be afraid to study the situation and act on it.

Your best nutritional bet is to eat the kind of diet recommended by the American Heart Association or the American Cancer Society – one that is low in saturated fats and calories and rich in fruits, vegetables and grains. If you would like to improve or change your diet, consider consulting a registered dietitian. A dietitian can help you alter your eating habits, whether your goal is to eat more nutritiously, gain or lose weight, or learn to prepare easy meals and snacks. The usual fee is about $75 for a one-hour consultation, which may be covered by your insurance. But the real change is up to you – no health professional can control what you eat.

"'Energy begets energy' used to be my mantra. 'Movement is life!' my message resounded. Now, the swelling in my joints tells me the truth. Movement is a gift.

"I want to exercise. I am sick and tired of my excuses for not being able to participate. Why can't I be the old, energy-packed me? Sure, my excuses are real. I am in my fifth year of rheumatoid arthritis. I have tried to cope with it and accept it. The flares are crippling and strike with no apparent reason. One day I am feeling well, the next day I have hot liquid burning in my joints. Cortisone injections into the offending joints are my only relief.

THE OTHER SIDE OF FITNESS
– MEREDITH BUNTING, VIRGINIA BEACH, VA

"I walk with swollen, cramped feet to greet members in the health club I have managed for 10 years. I direct them to the exercise equipment and tell them about energy-packed fitness classes – the ones I used to teach. As they press on, I slip back behind my wall of memories.

"On their way to exercise, my friends greet me. Their smiles touch me like rays of sunshine dispersing murky clouds. They treat me as if nothing has changed. Oh, they know I have had a 'setback.' But they believe in me. They don't pity me. They offer help and lend a hand. I begin to see another side of fitness: compassion.

"As I accept their help, I sense my walls crumbling. Letting go of what I can no longer do, inspired by the helping spirit of my friends, I feel a new source of energy. This side of fitness has great potential!"

Herbs, Supplements and "Natural" Remedies

These comprise the largest category of alternative therapies. Supplements such as herbs, minerals, animal extracts and enzymes – as well as more exotic remedies – are increasingly available to people with chronic health problems such as arthritis. What's more, people are buying and using them in record numbers. In 2004, a U.S. government study reported that 19 percent of U.S. adults use natural supplements.

Herbs, supplements and other such "natural" remedies have a tremendous attraction for people with arthritis who are frustrated with solutions offered by conventional medicine. Although most people realize no "magic bullet" can cure arthritis, they hope their pain and other symptoms will be better controlled if they add a supplement or extract to their prescribed medication.

Supplements offer the convenience of popping a pill or potion – and the belief that "natural" ingredients won't harm you. But natural doesn't always mean safe. Some people think that supplements – especially herbs – are safe because they are natural alternatives to the chemicals in prescription drugs. But herbs too are chemicals. And anything strong enough to help may also be strong enough to hurt.

We're not saying that supplements are bad. In fact, some extracts and supplements have been useful in treating various types of arthritis. For example, research shows that, taken in large quantities, the omega-3 fatty acids found in oils from certain fish modify inflammation associated with rheumatoid arthritis. Unfortunately, the effect may last only a few months. Another study showed that oil extracted from the borage plant had properties similar to nonsteroidal anti-inflammatory drugs (NSAIDs), without gastrointestinal side effects. However,

researchers have not yet determined effective dosages and possible long-term side effects of these supplements.

At this point, it is difficult to know the effect of supplements, in part because of a phenomenon known as the *placebo effect*. In many research studies, some people are given the actual pill or treatment being tested, while others unknowingly receive a placebo, an inactive pill or treatment. Some people taking the placebo will experience the same results (reduced pain, for example) as the people taking the real drug, pointing to the potency of the power of suggestion.

For most types of supplements, solid scientific evidence is not available. Few studies have been done to test supplements, and the studies that do exist usually don't stand up to rigorous scientific examination. In addition, the types of treatments are not regulated and tested in the same way that pharmaceutical products are to ensure that they are both safe and effective – and sometimes that's not even good enough. Witness the dangers of some COX-2 inhibitors, now off the market. Finally, few or no purity standards or quality control mechanisms are in place.

It may seem like a paradox, but most pills labeled "natural" contain processed chemicals, just as drugs do. It's true that "natural" substances are chemicals normally found in the body, while drugs are not. But chemicals in drugs are tested extensively for safety and purity, but those in "natural" pills are not tested to the same extent. It's fine to consider "natural" remedies, but you should be aware of the concerns.

If you do decide to try an herbal extract, dietary supplement or other "natural" remedy, proceed with caution and keep the following points in mind:

- **Ask questions.** Don't be afraid to ask your doctor, pharmacist or other health professionals for an opinion or a recommendation.
- **Buy wisely.** When purchasing a supplement, buy from a large company, pharmacy or health-food chain. They may have more stringent quality controls than small companies.
- **Read labels carefully.** No supplement can lawfully claim to treat, cure, diagnose or prevent disease. Look for products with the U.S.P. notation, indicating that the manufacturer followed standards established by the United States Pharmacopoeia, the public standards-setting authority for prescription and over-the-counter medicines, dietary sup-

plements, and other healthcare products manufactured and sold in the United States.

- **Try products one at a time.** If you try only one you can keep track of its effect (or lack of effect). If you notice side effects, stop taking the supplement right away.

COMMON SUPPLEMENTS USED FOR RA

Numerous herbs, supplements and similar treatments are touted as beneficial for people with rheumatoid arthritis. But do they really work or are they a waste of your money? In most cases, the treatments have not been scientifically tested to see if they are effective for RA symptoms. In other words, no solid evidence shows that they work – or even, in some cases, that they might not do more harm than good. They might be beneficial for some people but dangerous for others.

We urge you to be cautious when trying natural treatments like the ones listed below for RA. Why? Herbs and supplements are considered the same as food by the U.S. government. They may be sold without approval by the Food and Drug Administration (FDA) and, as we've noted, do not have the rigorous testing and sanctioning processes that drugs do.

Talk to your doctor before trying any herb or supplement about possible interactions with your current prescription or over-the-counter drugs. Do not rely on hearsay, or on the Web sites or literature of manufacturers or retailers that manufacture or sell the treatments.

For more information – including legitimate studies – on herbs and supplements, consult the Web site of the National Center for Complementary and Alternative Medicine, www.nccam.nih.gov, part of the National Institutes of Health. You can also find information about herbs and supplements used for arthritis on www.arthritis.org.

Black Currant Oil: Oil derived from the black currant seeds. Supposed to lessen RA joint pain, stiffness and swelling. Available in capsule form.

Borage Oil: Oil derived from the seeds of the borage plant. Supposed to lessen RA joint pain, stiffness and swelling. Available in capsule form.

Boron: Trace mineral found in many foods and multivitamins. Supposed to have anti-inflammatory effects and may improve joint and bone health. Available in many pill forms or in natural foods.

Boswellia: Gum resin from the bark of the Oswellia tree. Supposed to have anti-inflammatory effects and fight arthritis symptoms. Available in capsule or pill form.

Cat's Claw: Dried root bark of a Peruvian vine. Supposed to have anti-inflammatory effects. Available in many forms, including capsule, tablet and tea bag infusion.

Cayenne: Also known as *red pepper* or *capsaicin*, cayenne is a hot pepper whose oil is often used in topical creams. May temporarily relieve pain in small areas. Do not use with other heat sources, such as heating pads: that may cause burns. Not for internal use. Available in cream form.

Collagen: Protein found in human and animal cartilage. Supplement forms derived from animal only. Supposed to relieve pain, swelling, inflammation and stiffness. Available in capsule, tablet or powder form.

Curcumin: Pulverized root from the turmeric plant (the powder supplement is also called turmeric), commonly used in cooking. Supposed to relieve pain, inflammation and stiffness, and protect against memory loss. Available in capsule or powder form.

Devil's Claw: Plant found in southern Africa. Supposed to relieve pain and inflammation, as well as to aid digestion. Available in capsule, powder or tea leaf form.

Evening Primrose Oil: Seeds of a wildflower indigenous to America, containing gamma-linoleic (see below) acid. Supposed to lessen RA joint pain, stiffness and swelling. Available in capsule form.

Fish Oil: Oil derived from cold-water fish such as salmon, herring, tuna, mackerel and halibut, and cod (hence, the traditional treatment of cod-liver oil). Supposed to fight inflammation and morning stiffness, and reduce fatigue. Available in capsule or pill form, or by adding cold-water fish to diet.

Flaxseed: Seed of flax plant. Supposed to lessen stiffness and joint pain, and to "lubricate" joints. Available in seed, ground flour or meal, capsule or oil form.

Ginger: Dried or fresh root of *zingiber officinale* plant, or common gingerroot. Supposed to reduce inflammation and lessen joint pain, as well as protect the stomach from ulcers and the gastrointestinal side effects of NSAIDs. Available in powder, extract, tincture, spice and oil form.

GLA: Gamma-linoleic acid, an omega-6 fatty acid found in supplements like black currant oil, borage oil and evening primrose oil (see earlier listings). Supposed to have anti-inflammatory effects and to ease joint pain and stiffness. Available in capsule or oil form; must be taken orally.

MSM: Sulfur compound found in many fruits, vegetables and grains, and naturally occurring in animals and humans. Supposed to have anti-inflammatory and analgesic effects. Available in tablet and powder form, and can be taken orally or used topically.

Selenium: Essential mineral found in many multivitamins. Supposed to fight joint tenderness and pain, as well as inflammation. Can be toxic in larger doses than the body needs. Available in tablet form and in many multivitamins.

Stinging Nettle: Leaves and roots of the *urtica dioica* plant. Supposed to have anti-inflammatory effects and to ease aches and pains. Available in tea, tincture, extract or leaf form; can be used externally as a poultice.

Thunder God Vine: Roots and leaves of a vine found mostly in Asia, *tripterygium* *wilfordii.* Supposed to have anti-inflammatory and analgesic effects. May slow down an overactive immune system. Available in extract form.

Turmeric: See curcumin, page 155.

Willow Bark: Derived from the bark of the white willow tree. Contains *salicin,* an ingredient chemically similar to the active in ingredient in aspirin and many NSAIDs. Supposed to have anti-inflammatory and analgesic effects. Available in

Before Trying an Alternative Therapy

Many alternative therapies are not regulated.

Before you decide to try one of these therapies, find out as much as you can about it. A good source of information is the National Center for Complementary and Alternative Medicine (NCCAM), www.nccam.nih.gov. For a free packet of information, write to the NCCAM Clearinghouse, P.O. Box 7923, Gaithersburg, MD 20898-8218 or call 888-644-6226.

Once you have information on a particular therapy, discuss it with your doctor.

He or she will be able to answer questions such as "How will this affect my treatment plan ?" and "Could this cause problems by interacting with my medications?"

If you decide to proceed, do so with caution.

Seek out a qualified practitioner. For example, there are licensing requirements by state and/or national boards in biofeedback, acupuncture and massage therapy.

Consider the cost.

Many alternative therapies are expensive. Although physicians may recommend certain therapies such as massage, they may not be covered by your insurance policy.

Use good judgment.

If the practitioner makes unrealistic claims (such as, "This will cure your arthritis.") or suggests that you should discontinue your conventional treatment, do not continue with that practitioner.

Adapted from: *Kids Get Arthritis Too.* Atlanta: Arthritis Foundation. May/June 1999.

extract, tea or tincture form, as well as in some topical creams.

Zinc Sulfate: Mineral found in many multivitamins. Supposed to improve joint swelling, stiffness and overall well-being. Available in multivitamin compounds in liquid, capsule, softgel or tablet form, as well as in foods such as oysters, meat, eggs, tofu and black-eyed peas.

Prayer and Spirituality

Many people believe that prayer and spirituality can help us cope with suffering, offer comfort in times of illness and depression, and perhaps even help in healing. Public opinion polls have shown that prayer is one of the most commonly used alternative therapies for arthritis. Indeed, research in behavioral medicine suggests that the interactions of the mind, body and spirit can have powerful effects on our health. But very few published scientific studies have examined the effects of prayer and spirituality.

And it is difficult to measure the effects of prayer and faith on health. One way scientists have approached the issue is to compare people who regularly attend religious serviceswith others who do not. Such studies suggest that people who attend religious services tend to live longer, take bet-

ter care of their health and recover more quickly from illnesses and depression. However, skeptics contend that these studies really show the benefits of companionship and community, not religion.

People have found comfort, meaning and inspiration from prayer and other spiritual practices for thousands of years. Adding or deepening the spiritual aspects in your life could be good for you and arthritis, and – unless you abandon your medication and/or other components of your treatment program – certainly won't hurt you. But prayer alone will not "cure" your arthritis.

Miscellaneous Therapies

Many other types of alternative and complementary therapies are available. In fact, new ones seem to crop up every week. They range from the probably harmless (copper bracelets) to the potentially harmful (gin-soaked raisins). For a more in-depth look at therapies targeted to people with arthritis, check out *Alternative Treatments for Arthritis,* published in 2005 (see box on page 148).

Talking to Your Doctor About Your Options

Doctors are more willing than ever before to discuss the use of alternative and complementary therapies with their patients, in part because they realize that patients are using them, with or without a doctor's advice. Also, strong evidence suggests that many complementary therapies can and do relieve some of the symptoms of arthritis, at least in the short-term.

If your doctor seems reluctant to talk about alternatives to traditional medical treatment, don't give up. Tell your doctor that discussing the topic is important to you. Be insistent (but not confrontational). The following list of questions might help you open the lines of communication:

- Is this a therapy that might help my condition?
- Have you read any studies about or had experience with this type of therapy?
- Is this therapy controversial? Why (or why not)?
- What are the hazards of the therapy?
- Will there be any interaction between this therapy and the medications or other treatments you have prescribed for me?

- Where can I get more information on the therapy?

Remember, keeping your doctor informed about your treatment decisions is in your best interest. He or she can't give you the best professional advice without knowing all of the treatments you are using – whether they are over-the-counter drugs, herbal remedies or exercise programs.

Making Smart Choices

Now that you're better informed about the use of alternative and complementary therapies, become a smart consumer (see box, page 157). Be realistic when assessing the benefits and drawbacks of such therapies. Certain alternative/complementary practices can help ease some arthritis symptoms, improve your outlook and enhance the effects of your conventional arthritis treatment plan. However, the therapies cannot replace proven medical treatments, nor can they cure chronic disease.

PART THREE

Develop a Good Living Lifestyle

Chapter 14

Exercise:
The Importance of Getting Physical

If you have rheumatoid arthritis, you may think, "Exercise? Are you kidding? I don't have the energy or ability to even think about exercise!" But exercise is a very important component of RA management, and getting the right kind of exercise can make ordinary mobility easier and less painful.

Perhaps someone has told you that you should rest or protect your joints – and they're right. You do need to take extra care of joints that are actively inflamed. However, that does not mean you should avoid exercise. Believe it or not, it can also be an important way to protect your joints.

In this chapter, we will discuss some of the ways that regular exercise can benefit people with rheumatoid arthritis. We will also review the types of exercises that should be part of your routine and include some simple exercises to get you started.

Why exercise? Some kind of exercise is good for almost everyone, but research has shown that it can be especially helpful for people with rheumatoid arthritis. The disease process – and the damage it causes – may lead to limited joint range of motion, decreased muscle strength and endurance, and general deconditioning. Appropriate and regular exercise can lead to improvement in these areas; it also reduces pain, fatigue and depression. Some researchers have even shown that regular aerobic exercise can reduce joint swelling in people with rheumatoid arthritis.

What if I Don't Exercise?

When you're tired and your body hurts, you may not feel like exercising. It's all too easy to put off exercising because

Benefits of Regular Exercise

Keeps your body from becoming too stiff
Keeps your muscles strong
Keeps bone and cartilage tissue strong and healthy
Improves ability to do daily activities
Gives you more energy
Helps you sleep better
Helps control weight gain
Makes your heart stronger and improves cardiovascular health
Provides an outlet for stress and tension
Decreases depression and anxiety
Releases endorphins (your body's natural pain relievers)
Improves self-esteem and provides a sense of well-being

you're afraid that it will uses up the energy you need to complete your other daily activities. However, as the saying goes, "Use it, or lose it." Unused joints, bones and muscles deteriorate quickly. Long periods of inactivity can lead to weakness, stiffness, increased fatigue, poor appetite, constipation, increased blood pressure, obesity, osteoporosis, and heightened sensitivity to pain, anxiety and depression. Collectively, the results of inactivity are known as *deconditioning*. And, as the diagram here shows, deconditioning leads to further pain, in a continuing cycle.

How does the cycle work? If you do not exercise, your muscles become smaller and weaker, and they are less able to support and protect you. You have less stamina and daily activities become more difficult. The loss of function and independence can increase your level of stress, which in turn creates muscle tension, leading to more pain, and so on through the cycle.

Exercise is one of the prime weapons used to break this cycle. And studies show that regular exercise actually increases the amount of energy you have. Participating in a regular exercise program is a great way to feel better and move more comfortably with less pain.

Making a Commitment to Exercise

The idea of starting an exercise program can be intimidating, particularly if you've never been very active. Just keep in mind that you should start slowly. Do whatever you can at first. As you become stronger and your endurance increases, you will be able to exercise longer and more strenuously.

One of the toughest parts of exercise is getting started. But the effort you put into starting and maintaining a regular exercise program will reward you many times over in terms of better health, less pain and improved mental outlook. Once you begin to enjoy the benefits of exercise, your body will become more conditioned, and you will begin to look forward to your workouts.

The following list provides some ideas to help you get started and stay motivated. Use the ideas that make sense for your personality and situation.

• **Get a physical assessment.** See a doctor or physical therapist for an assessment of your exercise and joint protection needs. This will help you understand the reasons for exercise and set reasonable goals.

• **Set realistic exercise goals.** You may even sign a contract with yourself. Write down what you plan to do and when you plan to do it. You could have someone else "witness" the contract to help keep you motivated.

• **Make exercise a routine.** You may try to exercise at the same time each day so that it becomes a part of your routine. Try linking the time to something else: for example, after your morning shower, before lunch or after reading the newspaper.

• **Stay in the habit.** Do some exercise every day. Extra physical activity can add your physical conditioning. When you feel up to it, incorporate extra movement into your normal routines, such as walking up the stairs instead of using an elevator.

• **Make an effort every day.** On days that you have pain or you don't feel motivated, making some effort is important – even if you just do some gentle stretching or range of motion exercises.

• **Add variety.** Vary the type of exercises you do to keep from getting bored. Try doing some exercises, such as range of motion or muscle conditioning exercises, to music. Try rotating other exercises. For example, you could walk three days a week, swim twice and attend an arthritis exercise class twice. Ask a friend or family member to join you in a regular exercise routine. You can motivate each other, and make exercise social. If you make it fun, you'll be much more likely to stick with it.

• **Keep track of your progress and enjoy your successes.** There are many ways to monitor the effectiveness of your fitness program. Your doctor or health professional may notice decreased stiffness or improved gait. You will probably be able to see other benefits, such as less fatigue, less pain and decreased stress.

Choosing the Right Moves

We hope we've convinced you that exercise is important. But you may wonder what kinds of exercise you should include in your daily routine. People enjoy different types of exercises – and those with rheumatoid arthritis have a varying disease courses and levels of joint involvement, or inflammatory activity.

When you are starting out, your first contact may be with a health professional – a doctor, physical therapist, trainer or exercise therapist. He or she may have a list of recommended exercises and may give you explanatory diagrams. A complete exercise program to improve physical fitness may include exercises for flexibility, muscle strength and endurance, and cardiovascular fitness. How you combine these types of exercise depends on your current capacities, exercise experience, the goals you want to accomplish, and most of all, what you like to do. To

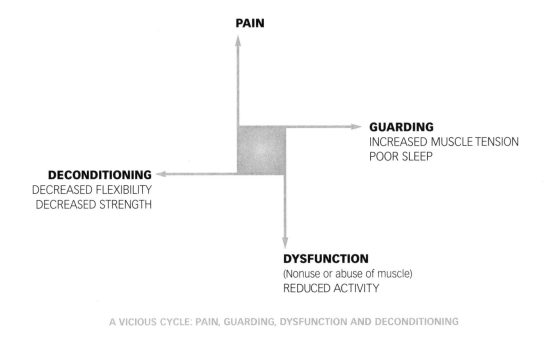

A VICIOUS CYCLE: PAIN, GUARDING, DYSFUNCTION AND DECONDITIONING

The Three Components of Total Fitness

Type	When To Do It	Potential Results
ROM or Flexibility	Every day As needed for better mobility As a warm-up or cool-down	Joint mobility Relaxation Make activity easier
Muscle Toning and Strength	Every other day for each muscle group With flexibility and aerobic exercises	Pain relief More energy Better endurance Makes activity easier
Endurance or Aerobic	Every day or as often as possible (at least three times weekly)	More energy Improved weight More stamina Lower blood pressure Better bone health

become a successful exercise self-manager, you need to discover which types of exercise are best for you and use them to meet your goals.

Flexibility (Stretching) Exercises

Flexibility exercises are intended to help keep your muscles stretched and your joints moving freely. They can be thought of as a foundation of your exercise program, because flexibility is necessary for comfortable movement during exercise and daily activities. It also helps reduce the risk of sprains and strains.

Flexibility exercises are also referred to as range-of-motion and stretching exercises. They should be done gently and smoothly, usually every day. You may be familiar with this type of exercise as a "warm up," because it is usually recommended before performing any more vigorous type of exercise.

If you have been inactive for a while, or if you have stopped exercising temporarily because of your arthritis, these exercises are a good way to begin your fitness program. You can start by building up to 15 minutes of flexibility exercises.

When you are able to do 15 continuous minutes, you should have the motion and endurance needed to begin adding strengthening and aerobic exercise to your program. Some sample flexibility exercises are included at the end of this chapter.

For people with rheumatoid arthritis, stiffness in the morning can be a big problem. Doing gentle flexibility exercises before getting up or during a hot bath or shower may help joints loosen up. However, doing them later in the day may be more comfortable for many people with rheumatoid arthritis and may reduce fatigue.

Strengthening Exercises

Exercises that increase muscle strength and endurance are the second important component of your fitness program. Joint swelling and pain can weaken muscles, as can disuse due to stiffness and pain. If you have arthritis, strong muscles are needed to climb stairs, walk safely, lift and

"As I sat in the New Orleans airport waiting for my sister to arrive, my heart was pounding. She had been diagnosed with rheumatoid arthritis two months before. The occasion of her visit was her 40th birthday, and I wanted this to be a joyous celebration. But I found myself feeling tearful as I waited for her plane to land. When I saw her, I breathed a sigh of relief. She didn't look any different, just slightly more somber.

RHEUMATOID ARTHRITIS FROM THE OUTSIDE: A SISTER'S VIEW
– BETH HODGENS, MACON, GA

"This was five years ago. I was fortunate enough to celebrate my sister's 45th birthday recently. She came to my hometown to play in a regional tennis championship. She and her partner blew their opponents away in the final match of the weekend.

"My sister is a single parent of two teenage boys and the director of marketing at a large hospital in Atlanta. Her motto has always been 'Keep moving.' Since her diagnosis with rheumatoid arthritis, that phrase has new meaning. Her ability to keep all the balls in the air, her attitude and her exercise have helped her gain a handle on her disease. She is a hero to me."

reach. Strong muscles are important to help absorb shock, support joints and protect you from injury.

Strengthening exercises (also called resistance exercises) make your muscles work harder by adding weight or resistance to movement. There are two types: isometric and isotonic. In isometric exercises, you tighten your muscles without moving your joints. This helps build the muscles around your joints. In isotonic exercises, you move your joints to strengthen your muscles. For example, straightening your knee while sitting in a chair is an isotonic exercise that helps strengthen your thigh muscle. Flexibility exercises can become strengthening exercises when you increase the speed, increase the number of repetitions, or add weight (resistance) to the exercise being done.

The goal of a good strengthening program is to work your muscles just enough to get them to adapt to the extra work by becoming stronger. This can be done by using hand-held or wrap-around weights, elastic bands or simply by using the weight of your body. Avoid working muscles so much that they are sore and stiff for a day or two after exercising.

If you have active inflammation, or if you need to protect certain joints, ask a therapist which strengthening exercises are

best and safest for you. If you have been inactive, start by doing 15 minutes of flexibility exercises before you attempt strengthening ones. Some sample exercises are illustrated at the chapter's end.

Endurance (Aerobic) Exercises

When you hear *aerobics,* do you think of young adults in skimpy clothes working up a sweat while loud music blares? Aerobic exercise means more than just aerobic dance. Also known as cardiovascular or endurance exercise, aerobic exercise is any physical activity that uses the large muscles of the body in rhythmic, continuous motions. Walking, dancing, swimming, bicycling or even raking leaves are all examples of aerobic exercise.

These exercises make up the third important part of your exercise routine. The purpose of aerobic exercise is to make your heart, lungs, blood vessels and muscles work more efficiently. This promotes overall health by reducing your risk of heart disease, high blood pressure and diabetes. For people with arthritis, aerobic exercise can improve endurance, strengthen bones, improve sleep, control weight, and reduce depression and anxiety.

Your fitness program should include aerobic activities three to four times each week. The goal is to work within your

Finding Your Target Heart Rate

To find your target heart rate, you must stop during your activity and take your pulse. Keep walking or moving around to keep your blood circulating. Placing your index and middle fingers on your opposite wrist or below your jawline at your neck, count your pulse for six seconds and add a zero to that number (or count for 10 seconds and multiply by six). For example, if you count 14 beats in a 10-second period, your heart rate is six times 14, or 84 beats per minute.

Using the chart for a guide, find the target heart rate for your age group. You don't want your heart rate to be faster than the top end of the range during your aerobic exercise. If it does exceed the maximum, slow it down. If you are a beginner, consider the higher number in your range as one you should not exceed. And take heart: if you exercise in your target range regularly, your endurance and conditioning will improve.

target heart rate for 30 minutes each session. If you are not able to exercise continuously for 30 minutes, work up to it slowly. Start with five minutes of gradually increasing activity, continue with five minutes of activity in your recommended heart range (see chart),

then decrease activity for five minutes. Once you are able to do that, you can increase the length of activity in your target range.

Walking. Walking is an excellent type of aerobic exercise for almost everyone. It requires no special skills and is inexpensive. You will need a good pair of supportive walking shoes, and you may need orthotics, or special shoe inserts. You can walk almost anytime and anywhere. Many towns now have mall walking clubs, providing a safe place to exercise whatever the weather outside.

Water exercise. Swimming and exercising in warm water are especially good for stiff joints and sore muscles. Water also helps support your body while you move your joints through their range of motion, placing little stress on your joints.

Bicycling. Cycling on a stationary bicycle is a good way to get aerobic exercise without placing much stress on your hips, knees or feet. Some stationary bicycles allow you to exercise your upper body as well. When beginning, try not to pedal faster than 15 to 20 miles per hour. As your fitness increases, you can up your speed and/or add resistance to your workout.

Rowing. Rowing on a machine – or if you are lucky enough, in a boat – is a good aerobic exercise for people with whose hips, knees or feet are affected by rheumatoid arthritis.

Ski machines. Cross-country skiing or using a machine that simulates that action is an excellent non-impact exercise. One of the least abrasive non-water exercises, it works both the upper and lower body.

A Note About Pain

You may be afraid to exercise too vigorously for fear of causing pain or damage to your joints– common concern for many people with rheumatoid arthritis. And you're right: gentle exercise is best. You can learn to tell the difference between pain you experience from sore muscles after exercising and pain caused by overuse or inflammation of joints.

Sore muscles are usually the result of overstretching or overuse after you have been inactive. This type of pain usually begins several hours after exercising and may

Recommended Heart Rate Ranges

Age	Heart Rate Range (60% - 75% of Age-Predicted Maximum Heart Rate)	10-Second Count
20	120 – 150	20 – 25
25	117 – 146	19 – 24
30	114 – 143	19 – 24
35	111 – 139	18 – 23
40	108 – 135	18 – 23
45	105 – 131	17 – 22
50	102 – 128	17 – 21
55	99 – 124	16 – 21
60	96 – 120	16 – 20
65	93 – 116	15 – 19
70	90 – 113	15 – 19
75	87 – 109	14 – 18
80	84 – 105	14 – 18
85	81 – 101	13 – 17
90	78 – 98	13 – 16

continue for 24 to 36 hours. If you experience muscle soreness, you may try spending more time doing flexibility or warm-up exercises before proceeding to more vigorous activity. You may want to scale back your program until your muscles become more accustomed to a certain level of exercise, then gradually increase your workout.

By contrast, swelling and pain may be a signal of overuse. If you notice these symptoms, you can treat the joint by elevating and resting it. You may need to modify your exercise program to avoid further stress to the joint.

One further note about pain: Exercise has been found to be one of the most consistently effective non-drug tools to reduce the pain associated with arthritis. So exercise sensibly, but do exercise. You will feel better.

Don't Go it Alone

Many people who exercise on their own find it hard to stay motivated and keep going. If you are among these people, it may help to exercise with at least one other person. Two or more people can keep each other motivated, and joining a class can give you a feeling of shared goals and camaraderie.

Most communities offer a variety of exercise classes, including special programs for people with arthritis, people over 50 or those who need adaptive exercises. The Arthritis Foundation sponsors exercise programs taught by trained instructors and developed specifically for people with arthritis. For information, contact your local chapter or branch office. Programs are also available through local YMCAs, health clubs, hospital-sponsored fitness facilities, community colleges, parks and recreation departments, and senior centers.

If you would like to join a community exercise class or health club, try to find one that meet your needs. Look for staff members who are certified by a professional organization, with training or experience in teaching exercise to people with arthritis or other special needs. The facilities – including the bathroom and changing areas – should be physically accessible. And you should feel comfortable with the staff and other members. Let your instructors know your concerns about special needs or modifications. If a facility does not offer you what you need, or you don't feel comfortable exercising there, find another one. If you don't enjoy exercising, you probably won't stick with it.

Sample Exercises

Here are some sample flexibility and strengthening exercises that you can try. Note the precautions, if any, and select the exercises that are best for you. You might check with your doctor first before beginning a new exercise program or routine if you are concerned. But most of the time, you are the best person to decide what exercises suit you. Use common sense and check with your doctor or therapist if you're not sure.

Neck Exercises

Purpose: Increase neck movement; relax neck and shoulder muscles; improve posture.

Precautions: Do these exercises slowly and smoothly. If you feel dizzy, stop the exercise. If you have had neck problems, check with your doctor before doing these exercises.

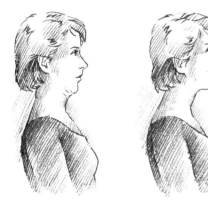
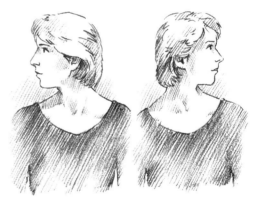

1. CHIN TUCKS

Pull your chin back as if to make a double chin. Keep your head straight – don't look down. Hold three seconds. Then raise your neck straight up as if someone was pulling straight up on your hair.

2. HEAD TURNS (ROTATION)

Turn your head to look over your shoulder. Hold three seconds. Return to the center and then turn to look over your other shoulder. Hold three seconds. Repeat.

Shoulder Exercises

Purpose: Increase mobility of the shoulder girdle (the bony structure that supports your upper limbs); strengthen muscles that raise shoulders; relax neck and shoulder muscles.

Precautions: If the exercise increases pain, stop and consult with your physician.

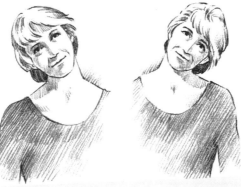

3. HEAD TILTS

Focus on an object in front of you. Tilt your head sideways toward your right shoulder. Hold three seconds. Return to the center, and tilt toward your left shoulder. Hold three seconds. Do not twist head but continue to look forward. Do not raise your shoulder toward your ear.

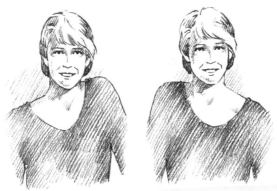

4. SHOULDER SHRUGS (ELEVATION)

(A) Raise one shoulder, lower it. Then raise the other shoulder; Be sure the first shoulder is completely relaxed and lowered before raising the other.

(B) Raise both shoulders up toward the ears. Hold three seconds. Relax. Concentrate on completely relaxing shoulders as they come down. Do not tilt the head or body in either direction. Do not hunch your shoulders forward or pinch shoulder blades together.

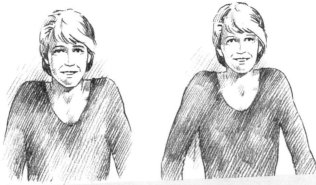

5. SHOULDER CIRCLES

Lift both shoulders up; move them forward, then down and back in a circling motion.

Then lift both shoulders up; move them backward, then down and forward in a circling motion.

Arm Exercises (Shoulders and Elbows)

Purpose: Increase shoulder and/or elbow motion; strengthen shoulder and/or elbow muscles; relax neck and shoulder muscles; improve posture.

Precautions: If you have had shoulder or elbow surgery, check with your surgeon before doing these exercises. These exercises are not advised for people with significant shoulder joint damage, such as unstable joints or total cuff tears.

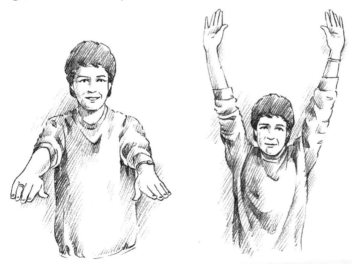

6. FORWARD ARM REACH

Raise one or both arms forward and upward as high as possible. Return to your starting position.

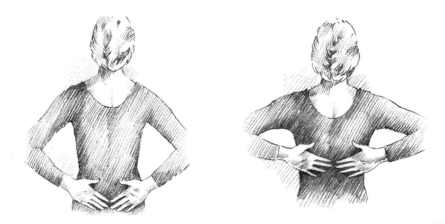

7. SELF BACK RUB (INTERNAL ROTATION)

While seated, slide a few inches forward from the back of your chair. Sit up as straight as possible; do not round your shoulders. Place the back of your hands on your lower back. Slowly move them upward until you feel a stretch in your shoulders. Hold three seconds, then slide your hands back down. You can use one hand to help the other. Move within the limits of your pain. Do not force.

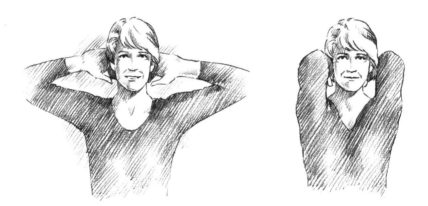

8. SHOULDER ROTATOR

Sit or stand as straight as possible. Reach up and place your hands on the back of your head. (If you cannot reach your head, place your arms in a "muscle man" position with elbows bent in a right angle and upper arm at shoulder level.) Take a deep breath in. As you breathe out, bring your elbows together in front of you. Slowly move elbows apart as you breathe in.

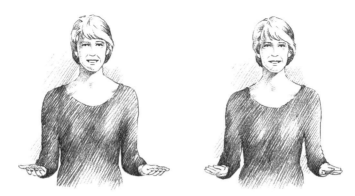

9. DOOR OPENER

Bend your elbows and hold them in to your sides. Your forearms should be parallel to the floor. Slowly turn forearms and palms to face the ceiling. Hold three seconds and then turn palms slowly toward the floor.

Wrist Exercises

Purpose: Increase wrist motion; strengthen wrist muscles.

Precautions: If you have had wrist or elbow surgery, check with your doctor before doing this exercise. Stop if you feel any numbness or tingling.

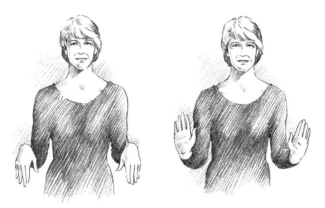

10. WRIST BEND (EXTENSION)

If sitting, rest hands and forearms on thighs, table, or arms of chair. If standing, bend your elbows and hold hands in front of you, palms down. Lift palms and fingers, keeping forearms flat. Hold three seconds. Relax.

Finger Exercises

Purpose: Increase finger motion; increase ability to grip and hold objects.

Precautions: If the exercise increases finger pain, stop and consult with your doctor.

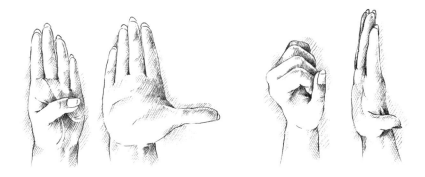

11. THUMB BEND AND FINGER CURL (FLEXION/EXTENSION)

(A) With hands open and fingers relaxed, reach thumb across your palm and try to touch the base of your little finger. Hold three seconds. Stretch thumb back out to the other side as far as possible. (B) Make a loose fist by curling all your fingers into your palm. Keep your thumb out. Hold for three seconds. Then stretch your fingers to straighten them.

Trunk Exercises

Purpose: Increase trunk flexibility; stretch and strengthen back and abdominal muscles.

Precautions: If you have osteoporosis or have had back compression fracture, previous back surgery or a hip replacement, check with your doctor before doing these exercises. Do not bend your body forward or backward unless specifically told to do so. Move slowly and immediately stop any exercise that causes you back or neck pain.

12. SIDE BENDS

While standing, keep weight evenly on both hips with knees slightly bent.

Lean toward the right and reach your fingers toward the floor. Hold three seconds. Return to center and repeat exercise toward the left. Do not lean forward or backward while bending, and do not twist the torso.

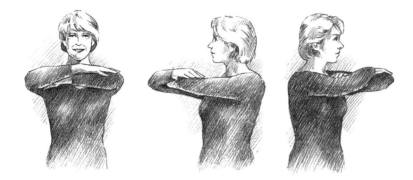

13. TRUNK TWIST (ROTATION)

Place your hands on your hips, straight out to the side, crossed over your chest, or on opposite elbows. Twist your body around to look over your right shoulder. Hold three seconds. Return to the center and then twist to the left. Be sure you are twisting at the waist and not at your neck or hips. NOTE: Vary the exercise by holding a ball in front of or next to your body.

Lower-Body Exercises

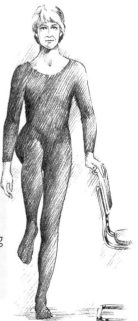

Purpose: Increase lower-body strength; increase range of motion in hip, knee and ankle joints.

Precautions: Check with your surgeon before doing these exercises if you have had hip, knee, ankle, foot or toe surgery, or any lower-extremity joint replacement. Do not rotate the upper body unless specifically told to do so. When standing, bend your knees slightly to avoid "locking" your knee joints.

14. MARCH (HIP/KNEE FLEXION)

Stand sideways next to a chair and lightly grasp its back. If you feel unsteady, hold onto two chairs or face the back of the chair. Alternating legs, lift them up and down as if marching in place. Gradually try to lift knees higher and/or march faster.

15. BACK KICK (HIP EXTENSION)

Stand straight on one leg and lift the other leg behind you. Hold three seconds. Try to keep your leg straight as you move it backward. Motion should occur only in the hip (not the waist). Do not lean forward – keep your upper body straight. NOTE: You can add resistance by using a large rubber exercise band around your ankles.

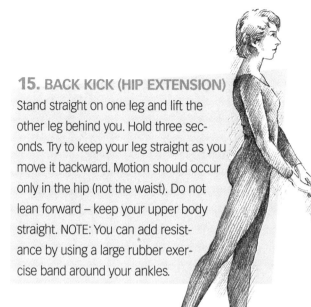

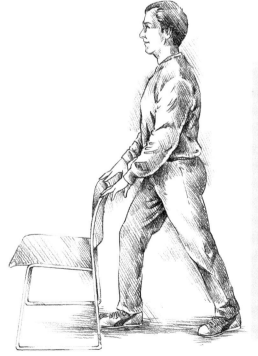

16. SIDE LEG KICK (HIP ABDUCTION/ADDUCTION)

Stand near a chair, holding it for support. Stand on one leg and lift the other leg out to the side. Hold three seconds and return your leg to the floor. Only move your leg at the top – don't lean toward the chair. Alternate legs.

Precautions: Check with your surgeon before doing these exercises if you have had a hip replacement. Keep the knee on the weight-bearing leg bent. Don't rotate your upper body; keep your chest and shoulders facing forward.

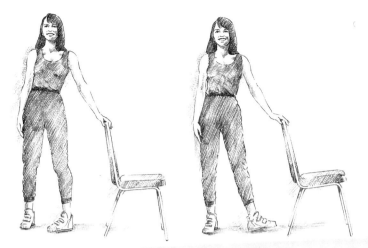

17. HIP TURNS (HIP INTERNAL/EXTERNAL ROTATION)

Stand with legs slightly apart, your weight on one leg and the heel of your other foot lightly touching the floor. Rotate your leg from the hip so that toes and knee point in and then out. Don't rotate your body; keep your chest and shoulders facing forward. NOTE: If you have difficulty putting weight on one leg, you can do this exercise by sitting at the edge of a chair with your legs extended straight in front and your heels resting on the floor.

Precautions: Check with your surgeon before doing these exercises if you have had a hip replacement. Don't rotate your upper body; keep your chest and shoulders facing forward.

18. SKIER'S SQUAT (QUADRICEPS STRENGTHENER)

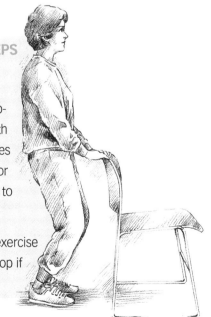

Stand behind a chair with your hands lightly resting on top of the chair for support. Keep your feet flat on the floor. With your back straight, slowly bend your knees to lower your body a few inches. Hold for three to six seconds, then slowly return to an upright position.

Precautions: Do not do the following exercise if you have had ankle or foot surgery. Stop if you experience calf pain or cramping.

19. TIPTOE (DORSI/PLANTAR FLEXION)

Face the back of a chair and rest your hands on it. Rise and stand on your toes. Hold three seconds, then return to the flat position. Try to keep your knees straight (but not locked). Now stand on your heels, raising your toes and front part of your foot off the ground. NOTE: You can do this exercise one foot at a time.

Precautions: If you have had recent ankle surgery, check with your surgeon before doing the following exercise.

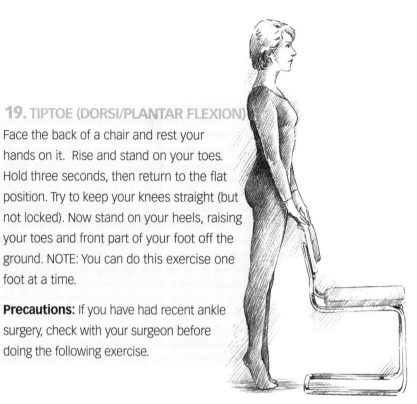

20. CALF STRETCH (GASTROCSOLEUS STRETCH)

Hold lightly to the back of a chair. Bend the knee of the leg you are not stretching so that it almost touches the chair. Put your other leg behind you, keeping both feet flat on the floor. Lean forward gently, keeping your back knee straight.

Precautions: Stop if the following exercises increase your back pain.

21. CHEST STRETCH (HIP EXTENSION AND PECTORALIS STRETCH)

Stand about two to three feet away from a wall and place your hands or forearms on the wall at shoulder height. Lean forward, leading with your hips. Keep your knees straight and your head back. Hold this position for five to 10 seconds, then push back to starting position. To feel more stretch, place your hands farther apart.

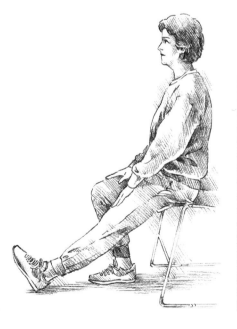

22. THIGH FIRMER AND KNEE STRETCH

Sit on the edge of your chair or lie on your back with your legs stretched out in front and your heels resting on the floor. Tighten the muscle that runs across the front of the knee by pulling your toes toward your head. Push the back of the knee down toward the floor so you also feel a stretch at the back of your knee and ankle. For a greater stretch, put your heel on a footstool and lean forward as you pull your toes toward your head.

Chapter 15

Eating Well:
Diet and Your Arthritis

Can what you eat cause, cure or affect your rheumatoid arthritis? Since symptoms of RA can vary from day to day, it's natural to think that what you ate yesterday may have caused or reduced the pain you feel today.

Research has not yet proven that any specific foods affect rheumatoid arthritis. But we do know that eating a good, balanced diet helps each body function at its best. Following a balanced diet can help you feel better, stay healthy, prevent chronic diseases such as some cancers and cardiovascular disease, and be a positive step toward managing your disease.

Adopt a Good Diet

Eating well does not mean you have to starve yourself or eliminate the foods you love. It means making gradual changes that allow you to focus on healthful meals you enjoy. You are more likely to stick with the changes listed below if you do them slowly:

- reduce salt, fat, cholesterol, sugar and alcohol intake
- include fiber, fruits and vegetables, and calcium-rich foods.

A Note on Diet "Cures"

You may read or hear about claims that special diets, supplements or foods cure health problems. Some of these claims are fraudulent. Others are unproven remedies (see Chapter 3). Consider diets unsafe and ineffective unless scientific tests prove them otherwise. Ask these questions:

- Does the diet eliminate any essential food group from the Food Guide Pyramid (discussed later in this chapter)?
- Does it stress only a few foods or eliminate certain foods?
- Does it claim to cure your arthritis?
- Are its ads misleading, created to look like news articles instead of advertising?

- Do its claims lack scientific evidence such as published studies?
- Do you suspect that the diet could be harmful to your health?

If the answer is yes to any of these questions, avoid the diet. If you do suspect that certain foods are related to any of your symptoms, discuss your concerns with your doctor.

What Is a Good Diet?

Experts recommend five basic guidelines for a balanced, healthful diet. Use these in planning daily meals. The following sections explain how each of the guidelines is helpful.

Eat a Variety of Foods

Variety, balance and moderation are keys to a healthful diet. Variety usually means eating more grains, fruits and vegetables than most Americans do. A good diet includes some choices from each of five different groups of foods: breads and cereals, fruits, vegetables, dairy products and meats. Together they provide the 40 or more nutrients your body needs to grow and function.

Pain, fatigue and depression can dampen your appetite or cause you to avoid foods that require time or effort to prepare. Follow the tips in the box below to make food preparation easier.

Health professionals in your community can help you learn more efficient cooking methods. For example, your doctor can refer you to an occupational therapist for advice on easier ways to cook. Some local chapters of the Arthritis Foundation and the cooperative Extension Services of some state universities also may sponsor cooking classes or demonstrations. In addition, the Arthritis Foundation publishes a free brochure called "Diet and Your Arthritis," which provides some basic guidelines for achieving a healthy overall diet. Call 800-568-4045 to order your free copy or visit the Arthritis Foundation Web site at www.arthritis.org to find your local chapter and receive other information.

Some medications can affect how well your body uses what you eat. For most people, eating a variety of foods will help boost nutrient levels. Ask your physician how your medications affect your nutrition and whether a vitamin supplement may be useful.

Ease up on Fat and Cholesterol

Reducing fats and cholesterol in your diet may help prevent cardiovascular disease. The American Heart Association recommends that people limit fat intake to no more than 30 percent of their calories –

and no more than 10 percent should be saturated fat. Someone eating 2,000 calories a day, for instance, should eat only 67 fat grams a day or less. AHA recommends a cholesterol intake of less than 300 milligrams per day, the equivalent of about one and a half eggs.

Fat, a source of concentrated calories, contributes to extra pounds. To lower saturated fat and cholesterol, choose low-fat meats and dairy products. Reduce servings of red meat and pork, and limit the use of added fats, oils, and salad dressings. A daily serving of red meat or pork the size of a deck of playing cards (approximately three ounces) is adequate for most adults.

Eat Vegetables, Fruits and Whole Grains

Carbohydrates are the basic energy supply for our bodies. Not all carbohydrates are equal, however. Simple carbohydrates, such as refined sugar and honey, contain few other nutrients. A candy bar will give you quick energy, but little else. We digest it quickly, which drives up blood sugar and strains our insulin-producing pancreas. The boost of energy received

Making Meal Preparation Easier

Pain can reduce your appetite and make meal preparation more difficult. You may tend to avoid foods that take more time and effort to prepare. Here are a few ways that you can make meal preparation easier on your body so that it is easier to eat healthfully.

- Plan rest breaks during meal preparation.

- Use good posture to avoid pain during cooking tasks.

- Arrange your kitchen for convenience. Keep the tools you use most within easy reach.

- Buy healthy convenience foods such as sliced and chopped vegetables.

- Add fresh fruit and bread to a frozen dinner for a simple, satisfying meal.

- Use kitchen appliances and tools that save time and effort, such as electric can openers and microwave ovens.

- Share meals with friends or family members so you can split the cooking tasks and enjoy the company.

by our bodies after eating candy bars doesn't last long.

Complex carbohydrates – fruits, vegetables and whole-grains like high-fiber rolls – are digested more slowly, are low-fat and create a feeling of fullness, a help to any weight watcher. (Overeat either form of carbohydrate, however, and your body converts the excess to fat.) Eat a slice of whole wheat bread, for example, and you get energy but also vitamins, minerals, fiber and some protein. Fiber comes from parts of plants your body cannot digest. Some types of fibers result in softer stools, less constipation and more rapid elimination of waste. Fibers such as oat bran also help lower cholesterol levels. Fiber from foods is preferable to fiber from supplements, because you get the additional nutrients in foods like bran, fruits and vegetables.

Spare the Sugar and Salt

Too much sugar adds excess calories and promotes weight gain and tooth decay. When checking food labels for added sugar, look for the words *dextrose, sucrose, fructose, honey* and *dextrin*. Carbohydrates should make up 55 percent to 60 percent of your calories, and the bulk should come from complex carbohydrates such as vegetables, fruits and grains.

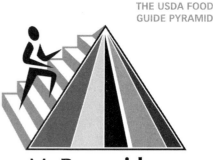

The American Heart Association suggests that you hold sodium intake to about 2,700 mg a day, or about 1 1/4 teaspoon of salt. Sodium causes your body to retain water and can affect your blood pressure. Many foods now come with low- or no-salt-added choices, which makes it easier to maintain a low-sodium diet. Watch for excess sodium levels on prepared food labels.

Drink Alcohol in Moderation

Excessive alcohol consumption can have adverse effects on your health, including weakened bones, which can lead to osteoporosis. Alcohol adds unwanted pounds with extra, empty calories. It can also increase the uric acid in the body, upping your susceptibility to gout marked by pain and inflammation.

Alcohol does not mix well with certain medications used in treating rheumatoid arthritis. Stomach problems also are more likely if you drink alcohol and take aspirin or other nonsteroidal anti-inflammatory drugs (NSAIDs). Large amounts of alcohol combined with acetaminophen can damage the liver. If you are taking any medications, check with your doctor or pharmacist about drinking alcohol, even in moderation.

The Food Guide Pyramid

The Food Guide Pyramid, developed by the U.S. Department of Agriculture, shows how to follow healthy dietary guidelines and make wise food choices. Select most foods from the bottom two layers of the pyramid and fewer foods from the top, based on the recommended number of servings. The pyramid can guide you to a balanced diet with moderate amounts of sugar, sodium and saturated fat, and the right amount of calories to maintain a healthy weight.

The Food Labeling Act

With the Food Labeling Act of 1994, manufacturers of food products were required to provide a new, more comprehensive nutrition label on their packaging. Many products already listed ingredients, but there were no standards for comparing one food with another. The new labels allow you to evaluate the nutritional content of the food so you can make smart choices for a healthier diet.

The Food Labeling Act also set new guidelines for what health claims a food manufacturer can make. Claims such as "fat-free," "cholesterol-free," "low-sodium," and others are now defined by government standards. Manufacturers must meet certain requirements to make the claims. Instead of learning what each claim means, remember these key words to help you judge nutritional content:

- **Light:** A food has one-third fewer calories or half the fat of the standard version of the food (for example, light potato chips would have half the fat of standard potato chips). The sodium content of a low-calorie, low-fat food is reduced by 50 percent.
- **Low:** You can eat a large amount of this food without exceeding the daily value for the particular nutrient that is described as "low."
- **Fat-free:** The item contains less than 0.5 grams of fat per serving.
- **A fat-free food:** The food naturally has no fat.
- **Lean:** The fat content of meat is less than 10 grams of fat, less than 4 grams of saturated fat, and less than 95 milligrams of cholesterol per serving and per 100 grams.

- **Extra-lean:** The fat content of meat is less than 5 grams of fat, less than 2 grams of saturated fat, and less than 95 milligrams of cholesterol per serving and per 100 grams.
- **High:** One serving of the food contains 20 percent or more of the daily value for the nutrient being described (such as calcium).
- **Good source:** One serving of the food contains 10 percent to 19 percent of the daily value for the nutrient being described.

Nutrition Resources

Many information resources can answer your questions about your diet. One place to start is with your doctor. He or she can refer you to experts in diet and nutrition for help with applying diet guidelines, planning a weight-loss program or answering any of your questions.

Here are some other tips:

- Check with local hospitals, health clinics and public health departments, which often have individual nutritional counseling and weight-reduction groups.
- Search for a registered dietitian or a nutritionist in the Yellow Pages of the telephone directory or by asking your doctor.
- Go to www.MyPyramid.gov for information on the food guide pyramid. Or write USDA Center for Nutrition Policy and Promotion, 3101 Park Center Drive,Room 1034, Alexandria, VA 22302-1594.
- Contact the Cooperative Extension Service for answers to your questions about meal planning. Look under the "Government Offices" section of your phone book.
- Contact other voluntary health and professional organizations that promote a healthy diet, such as local chapters of the American Heart Association, American Cancer Society, American Diabetes Association and American Dietetic Association.
- Check your bookstore or library for relevant, recently published books on diet, weight loss or general nutrition.

PART FOUR

Assume Responsibility for What You Can Control

Chapter 16

Closing the Gates:
Ways to Manage Pain

Having rheumatoid arthritis can create many physical challenges in your daily life. Although treatments for arthritis have improved dramatically in recent years, dealing with daily morning stiffness or occasional flares can seem daunting. Also, you may wonder what you can do to save wear and tear on your joints.

In this chapter, we will discuss some tips and techniques to help you deal with the physical side of rheumatoid arthritis: acute and chronic pain, as well as the physical limitations that can result from stiffness and joint damage.

Your overall program for managing rheumatoid arthritis contributes to lessening pain. So, committing yourself to regular exercise, balancing activity with rest, and respecting your limits are important. You are not giving in to your pain; rather, you are finding ways to manage it.

Pain from rheumatoid arthritis may have several causes and solving the problem different approaches.

- **Inflammation.** This process causes your joints to swell and become red.
- **Damage to joint tissues.** Damage may be due to the disease process of rheumatoid arthritis, or from stress or pressure on the joints.
- **Muscle tightness or fibromyalgia.** Inflammation of the joints may at times lead to muscle weakness or stiffness. Some people with rheumatoid arthritis also experience fibromyalgia, marked by widespread muscle pain.

Fatigue and poor sleep – both of which are common in people with rheumatoid arthritis – amplify pain. Feelings of depression or psychological helplessness can lower your pain threshold, making you more vulnerable to pain.

Although you are no stranger to pain, it doesn't have to dominate your life. Most people experience good and bad days. Pain management specialists emphasize that a healthy approach to coping with pain can help you make the most of your good days and minimize the pain you feel on bad ones. Whether dealing with acute pain during a flare or ongoing, everyday pain, you can learn to help yourself by thinking about your relationship to pain and applying some of the techniques in this chapter that appeal to you.

One woman with rheumatoid arthritis says that she has learned to remind herself during pain episodes that her body is sick, but her mind is not. By using your mind – to implement relaxation techniques or to organize daily chores more efficiently – you can become your own best ally in managing pain.

What Is Pain?

When your body is injured in any way, the nerves of your damaged tissue trigger the release of chemicals. These chemicals relay messages to your brain, causing the unpleasant sensations we call pain. The many causes of pain are range from inflammation to trauma. Pain may be sharp or dull, chronic or acute, localized (felt in only one or two places) or general-

ized (felt throughout the body). In rheumatoid arthritis, pain may be caused by *synovitis*, or inflammation of the synovial membrane surrounding the joint. The result is swelling and tenderness.

Individual responses to pain vary. What one person can barely feel, another can hardly tolerate. This is one reason your doctor must rely on your reports of pain when examining you and when prescribing pain medications. Pain can be measured on various scales, such as a visual analogue scale, which asks you to rate your pain on a scale of 0 to 10 (or 0 to 100), with zero indicating no pain and 10 (or 100) indicating severe pain. Keeping track of your pain scores can help you and your doctor see how your disease is progressing and whether your pain medications and coping strategies are working.

The "Gate" Theory of Pain

Your nervous system plays an important role in how you experience pain. You may have heard reports about people with traumatic injuries who feel no pain immediately after the accident. The nervous system blocks the pain signals by producing chemicals called *endorphins* that lead to a good feeling. Other situations can trigger production of endorphins; for instance, runners often experience a "runner's high," or euphoria, during their runs.

So why is it that some pain signals get blocked? According to one theory, known as the gate control theory of pain, when pain signals reach the nervous system, they stimulate a group of nerve cells that form a "pain pool." When the cells reach

Non-Drug Strategies for Closing the Gate on Pain

- **Hot and cold treatments.** Usually applied directly to the pain site, heat may be more useful for chronic pain, and cold packs provide relief from acute pain.

- **Positive attitude and thoughts.** Consciously switching to positive thoughts can distract your brain from feeling pain.

- **Exercise.** Keeping your joints and muscles moving helps improve your general fitness level and can decrease pain.

- **Relaxation techniques.** You can train your muscles to relax and your thoughts to slow down by using these techniques, which include deep breathing, guided imagery and visualization, among others.

- **Massage.** Done properly, the method can relax your muscles and help you let go of tension.

- **Electrical stimulation.** Also called transcutaneous electrical nerve stimulation (TENS), the therapy is delivered through a small device that sends a painless electrical current to large nerve fibers, generating heat that relieves stiffness and pain. The current also stimulates the release of endorphins, the body's natural pain killers. TENS is usually prescribed by your doctor or physical therapist.

- **Topical lotions.** These are applied directly to the skin over the painful muscle or joint. They may contain salicylates or capsaicin, which decrease sensitivity to pain.

- **Acupuncture.** Considered a complementary or nontraditional therapy, acupuncture is the practice of inserting fine needles into the body along special points called "meridians" to relieve pain (see Chapter 13 on complementary and alternative therapies).

- **Sense of humor.** Many studies have demonstrated that humor can bolster the immune system and increase the ability to handle pain.

a certain level of activity, a virtual gate opens up, allowing the pain signals to proceed to higher centers in the brain. However, the gate can also be closed by certain signals. For example, medications such as morphine and other narcotics act as synthetic endorphins blocking the pain signal, so the gate does not open.

Research has shown that, in addition to pain medication, nondrug factors can be used to close the pain gate. Some or all of the strategies listed in the box on this page may help you deal with your pain. Many of them are discussed at greater length in this chapter or the chapters that follow, as well as in *The Arthritis Foundation's Guide to Pain Management,* available by calling 800-283-7800 or online at www.arthritis.org.

Pain experts now believe that the process of chronic pain may be more complex than that of acute pain. People with chronic pain may experience actual physical changes in the various nerves that receive and transmit pain signals, causing pain to continue even when the actual stimulus or cause of the pain (such as inflammation) is not there. So in RA and other chronic diseases, you may have to treat the pain as well as its underlying cause. New treatments, including implants, electronic stimulation devices,

and time-released drugs, may help in some cases. But you can also do a great many things – including those suggested in the box on page 197 – to manage your own pain.

Knowing what narrows the pain gate can help you feel more in control and create a plan of action to deal with pain. However, you should be aware that, just as certain factors can close the pain gate, others can open it, making you feel more pain. Some of these factors, such as a flare, are beyond your control. But you can control other factors, at least in part. These include:

- Prolonged stress or anxiety.
- Obsessing about pain and having negative thoughts.
- Too little physical activity.
- Too much physical activity or exertion.
- Overindulgence in alcohol.
- Overuse of pain medications.

Why "Grin And Bear It" Doesn't Work

There may be times when you think that the best strategy for dealing with pain is to simply ignore it. Although this approach may work for short periods – say, as you override pain in your hands to finish typing a document or ignore hip pain to dance at your friend's daughter's wedding – it is rarely wise to ignore or deny pain for long periods. If you are reluctant to admit pain to yourself or your doctor, or request medications, remember that pain is a signal that something is not right inside your body.

Research suggests that chemicals released by your body when you are feeling pain can actually make the inflammation of rheumatoid arthritis worse. The only good thing about pain is that it signals you something is wrong. Feeling pain over long periods has no advantage. Don't be afraid to take medications to relieve your pain.

Just because others cannot see your pain, does not mean you are not justified in addressing it. If you have concerns about becoming dependent on pain medication, speak to your doctor. Most drugs prescribed for pain relief are not addictive, and even potentially addictive drugs usually do not lead to chemical dependence in people who experience severe pain.

Managing a Flare

Although rheumatoid arthritis is a chronic disease, you can have acute episodes of pain and inflammation, known as flares. Flares may occur after infections, or after highly stressful situations. Often, however, what triggers a flare is not clear. You may have long periods when your rheumatoid

Warming Techniques

- Take a long and very warm shower first thing in the morning to ease morning stiffness.

- Soak in a warm bath or whirlpool.

- Buy a moist heat pad from the drugstore, or make one at home by putting a wet wash cloth in a freezer bag and heating it in the microwave for one minute. Wrap the hot pack in a towel and place it over the affected area for 15 to 20 minutes.

- To soothe stiff and painful joints in your hands, apply mineral oil to your hands, put on rubber dishwashing gloves, and place your hands in hot tap water for 5 to 10 minutes.

- Incorporate other warming elements into your daily routines, such as warming your clothes in the dryer before dressing or using an electric blanket and turning it up before getting out of bed.

A physical therapist can give you many additional ideas for using heat to relieve pain temporarily and ease stiffness.

arthritis is quiet, or in remission. Then, suddenly, the inflammation becomes more active and you have an arthritis flare.

Flares can be alarming, not only because of the pain, but because their timing is unpredictable. You may feel discouraged or afraid of further damage to your joints. You sometimes wonder whether something you did caused the flare.

What can you do to combat these feelings? Remember that you have a range of tools in your arsenal to address pain – from asking your doctor to increase your pain medications to applying cold packs or practicing deep breathing techniques. Also, remember that flares do calm down. You may want to think about how you will handle the inevitable bad days and flares before you experience them. Preparing for a flare can help you jump into action when it happens.

Personally Speaking STORIES FROM REAL PEOPLE

"In 1994, I noticed a strange soreness and stiffness in my hands, then in my wrists and ankles. In less than a year, every joint was engulfed in pain. I found it difficult to continue the simple tasks of living – caring for myself and my family, sleeping, working. They all became almost impossible. It hurt just to move. I was living, but I did not feel alive. To control the pain, I was on many medications, some with dangerous side effects.

I CALL IT MY CHRISTMAS GIFT
– STACY WHITE-WERNER, PERRY, MI

"Despite medications and therapies, I continued to get worse. Then, in December 1998, I started taking the drug *Enbrel*. I call it my Christmas gift. I have been on this medication since then, and the results are fantastic. I am not in remission, but I am close. I feel stronger every day. I am slowly getting my life back. I am continuing the education that I had put off. I feel like a wife and mother again. When I can completely control my symptoms, I plan on returning to work.

"In addition to medications, I also try to stay active and eat a well-balanced diet. My friends and family are also part of my healing process. Without their love and support, it would be tough to face life with rheumatoid arthritis. They give me the added strength to keep living in spite of it. The other way I cope is by keeping a positive outlook. This is my life and my body. I'm not going to let rheumatoid arthritis steal any more away from me."

Discuss a plan of action with your doctor. One approach would be to adjust your medications temporarily while the disease is unusually active. This will not only relieve some of the pain associated with a flare, but also help minimize any damage that may occur from unchecked inflammation.

Be aware that your medications may not control the flare right away, even if your dosages are increased. Or they may only have a limited effect on your flare. Of course you and your doctors should be in agreement about possible increases in your medications, or even additions of new medications during a flare. Many doctors will suggest a plan that you can use at each flare's onset without having to seek his or her permission each time.

The following is a list of some other steps that you may want to incorporate in your plan. Remember, some techniques work better for some people than others. Try a few of these, and if they don't work for you, discard them and try others.

• **Balance periods of activity with periods of rest.** Although more rest can help during a flare, you probably do not need to abandon your regular activities, work or exercise program. A doctor or physical therapist can help you modify your program when you experience a flare. Spending long periods in bed is counterproductive, usually prolonging your pain. Instead, try to intersperse periods of rest with some light activity. Finally, to keep joints from becoming stiff, move them through the fullest range of motion possible, gradually increasing your range as the flare subsides.

• **Have a plan to deal with your obligations.** Have a contingency plan both for work and family obligations. At work, try to arrange for coverage, work fewer hours per week or bring work home. Discuss your plan with supervisors and co-workers ahead of time, and assure them of your commitment. At home, plan to apportion a few extra jobs among family members, and make sure everyone knows what they are expected to do to keep things running smoothly.

• **Communicate with your family and friends.** The time to let your family and friends know that you may need more help is when things are going well. When a flare occurs, if someone volunteers to help you, give them a specific job. Otherwise, well-intentioned offers of assistance go unused. Other sources of help such as members of your religious institution or community volunteer organizations may be available to you as well.

• **Apply a hot or cold pack to inflamed joints.** Some people find hot or cold packs helpful. Although heat can theoretically make inflammation worse, because it tends to increase blood flow and nerve sensitivity, some people find a warm pack soothing and pain relieving. Others get great benefit form cold, which decreases blood flow to the inflamed area and decreases inflammation and muscle spasm, providing temporary relief from acute pain. You can buy warm and cold packs from a drugstore or medical supply outlet, or you can use a hot water bottle or simply wrap a towel around a bag of frozen vegetables (to avoid ice burn, never place the ice pack directly on your skin). The pack should be comfortable to the contours of the joint. Leave the pack on the area for about 10 minutes, then remove it for an equal amount of time. Some people even prefer warm packs for certain joints and cold packs for others. You will learn your own preferences through trial and error.

• **Practice relaxation or mind-diversion techniques.** These techniques work best when you practice them on a regular basis. Even though relaxation may not directly reduce your pain, it can minimize stress, which is a factor shown to amplify pain.

Many other techniques are available. When you find those that work for you, write them down and use them as often as needed – particularly when you experience a bad day or a flare.

Managing Chronic Pain

Chronic pain – defined as pain that lasts longer than a few months – can be even more challenging to deal with than acute pain. You probably know from experience that a flare does not last, and you will feel better. However, handling the chronic pain and stiffness that go on day after day can lead to fatigue, discouragement and even depression. For some people with rheumatoid arthritis, pain becomes a constant companion. Learning to manage your chronic pain is important so that you do not become its victim.

Some of the techniques that work for acute flares, such as relaxation, meditation and guided imagery, are also helpful in reducing or minimizing chronic pain. One goal of these approaches is to train your brain and body to focus on positive and pleasing images, directing your attention away from your pain. The beneficial effects seem to build over time, so practicing them regularly is important for good results.

In addition, treatments involving heat or cold can provide soothing relief for stiff joints and tired muscles. There are many forms of these therapies. You can experiment with the warming ideas in the box on this page to find which ones work best for you.

Avoiding Joint Pain And Damage

To manage pain well requires acting without waiting it to become severe. The same is true for managing joint damage: you can reduce the day-to-day stresses placed on joints in everyday activities.

In addition to regular exercise, you can learn ways to use your body to reduce joint stress. You can avoid trying to open tight-fitting jars and performing twisting motions on the dance floor. Learning to listen to your body's signals when you need to rest can also reduce pain, because energy reserves enhance your abilities to cope with pain. Some common techniques are described here, along with examples.

Body Mechanics or Ergonomics

Body mechanics is the use of proper techniques for bending, lifting, reaching, sitting and standing. The idea is always to use the largest and most stable joints to do the work. This spreads out the load and lessens stress on weaker joints, or those with more disease involvement.

- **Use your palms.** When you lift or carry things, use the palms of both hands instead of your fingers.
- **Use large muscles.** If you carry a purse, put it over your shoulder or consider switching to a back pack or fanny pack.
- **Lift with your legs.** When lifting something low or on the ground, always bend your knees and lift by straightening your legs.
- **Stand up properly.** To get up from a chair, slide forward to the chair's edge and place your feet flat on the floor. Lean forward, then push down with your palms (not your fingers) on the arms or seat of the chair. Stand up by straightening your hips and knees.
- **Practice good posture.** When standing, practice good posture by imagining a straight line that connects your ears, shoulders, hips, knees and heels. Knees should be slightly bent, stomach and buttocks tucked in, and shoulders back.
- **Use props.** Put some pillows on a chair, and consider using a raised toilet seat, to help you get up and down more easily.

Balancing Rest and Activity

Both work and leisure activities are important – the trick is balancing them. Moderation should be your motto, especially when your arthritis is more active.

- **Pace yourself.** Take short breaks, and alternate heavy and light activities during the day.
- **Don't set unrealistic goals.** Make a "To Do" list that isn't too long – and don't add to it.
- **Keep active.** Too much rest is not good for your joints either. Even on days when you are tired or stiff, try to do some exercise. By increasing your level of fitness, you will have more energy and less pain.
- **Know when to take breaks.** Don't wait for the physical signals of pain before you rest.

Organize and Simplify Your Life

We would all like to be more organized and able to streamline our daily routines. It's an especially good idea if you have rheumatoid arthritis, because the energy you save at work, for example, by having everything you need within reach may mean the difference between coming home exhausted and being able to enjoy the evening. Your health professional may offer some guidance to help you organize your life, but you can get started by using a few simple ideas.

- **Keep tools handy.** If you work, keep all equipment and tools within easy reach and at a comfortable level. Use a lazy Susan or storage bins to keep supplies accessible.
- **Simplify cleaning.** Streamline cleaning chores by using some of the new "all in one" cleaning products, or those that require little or no scrubbing. Don't try to clean everything in one day – rotate the tasks over the course of the week instead.
- **Plan ahead.** When cooking, put all necessary tools and ingredients on the counter before you start to minimize trips to the pantry and refrigerator. Use convenience foods – such as chicken that is precooked and cubed – to save energy and wear and tear on joints.
- **Organize your errands.** If your bank is near the dry cleaner, make one trip instead of two.

Self-Help Devices

When you're tired, stiff or in a hurry, self-help devices can make tasks easier on your joints and more efficient for you. The products, which range from simple to elaborate, help keep joints in the best position for functioning, provide leverage when needed, and extend your range of motion. The companies listed in the accompanying box are some of the many that sell self-help devices. Simple devices, such as jar openers, reachers and easy-grip utensils can be purchased at many hardware or medical supply stores.

- **In the bedroom.** When dressing, zipper pulls and buttoning aids can help you fasten clothing. Or you can choose to wear clothing with Velcro fasteners when available. A long-handled shoehorn extends your reach without bending.

- **In the kitchen.** In the kitchen, appliances such as electric can openers, food processors and mandolins (for slicing) make work easier. Reachers (long-handled tools with a gripping mechanism) can be used to retrieve items stored high or low. Built-up handles and grips make utensils easier to grasp and put less stress on finger joints. Install a fixed jar opener, or keep a rubber jar opener in the kitchen.

- **In the bathroom.** Tub bars and handrails provide additional stability and security when you are getting into and out of the bath or shower. These are a must if you have problems with balance. Faucet levers or tap turners are available if your grip is weak. A raised toilet seat can make it easier to sit down and get up from the toilet.

- **In the office.** In the work environment, many devices and modifications are available, from chairs and work surfaces with adjustable-height to telephones with large push buttons and hands-free headsets. If you are facing work modifications, you will probably want to see an occupational therapist. He or she can help you make changes and obtain the devices you need.

- **At play.** Leisure activities can still be enjoyable through the use of assistive devices such as kneelers and light-weight hoses for gardening, "no-hands" frames for quilting or embroidery, and card holders and shufflers for card games.

- **In the car.** When driving, a wide key holder can make it much easier to turn on the ignition. A gas cap opener can help when filling the tank at the gas station.

Where to Purchase Self-Help Devices

The companies listed below are manufacturers of ergonomic office equipment and daily living equipment. You may request catalogs and purchase directly from the company or through your physical therapist, occupational therapist or health care provider.

This list is by no means complete, but it may give you a good place to begin searching for useful products. Consult a physical or occupational therapist, or speak to your doctor, to find more sources of self-help or assistive devices. The Arthritis Foundation chapter near you may be able to give you more information on where to find helpful devices and can give you a copy of the Arthritis Today Buyer's Guide, a publication that lists a variety of helpful products, services and retailers.

The non-profit Illinois Assistive Technology Program helps people find assistive devices and maintains lists of companies that sell them. The organization can provide information specific to your state:

Illinois Assistive Technology Program
1 West Old State Capitol Plaza, Suite 100
Springfield, IL 62701
800-852-5110 (in Illinois Only)
217-522-7985
www.iltech.org

Ergonomic Office Equipment

Ergonomic Solutions
129 N. Sylvan Drive
Mundelein IL 60060-4949
800-755-4950
www.goergo.com
Call to obtain their catalog of products, including the Ergo rest and other arm supports, to make computer keyboarding easier.

Ergo Source
P.O. Box 695
Wayzata, MN 55391
404-952-1969
www.ergosource.com
To receive their information, leave a message requesting company literature. Products include office accessories, forearm supports, foot rests and adjustable work surfaces.

Daily Living Equipment

Sammons Preston Rolyan
Patterson Medical Company
P.O. Box 5071
Bolingbrook, IL 60440
800/558-8633
www.sammonspreston.com
Upon request, the company will send you their "Enrichment" catalog.

North Coast Medical

Consumer Products Division
18305 Sutter Blvd.
Morgan Hill, CA 95037
800-235-7054
www.ncmedical.com
NCM offers catalogs featuring products to help with everyday living and workplace needs.

Aids for Arthritis, Inc.

35 Wakefield Drive
Medford NJ 08055
800-654-0707
www.aidsforarthritis.com
Leave a message with your name and address, and the company will send you their "Self Help Products" catalog.

Sears Health and Wellness Catalog

7700 Brush Hill Road, Suite 240
Burr Ridge, IL 60527
800-326-1750
www.searshealthandwellness.com
Although Sears does not offer a separate catalog for people with arthritis, they will send you a copy of their health and wellness product catalog.

Kinsman Enterprises

10804 Mark Twain Road
West Frankfort, IL 62896-4105
618-9332-3838
www.kinsmanenterprises.com
This company manufactures products to help people do everyday tasks more easily. Contact the company for information about where to buy the products.

Chapter 17

Feeling Exhausted:
How to Cope with Fatigue

Fatigue is one of the most common symptoms experienced by people with rheumatoid arthritis – and sometimes the first sign of inflammation. During periods of inflammatory activity, feeling overwhelmingly fatigued, with no energy is not unusual. This overwhelming fatigue can impair your ability to concentrate, make you less able to deal with pain, and increase your feelings of helplessness. Like pain, fatigue is a signal that something is wrong. Pay attention to this signal.

Fatigue may be caused by several factors including inflammation, overdoing routine activities, medication side effects, stress and depression. Poor sleep and nutrition, and absence of regular exercise also may increase feelings of fatigue.

Feeling tired all the time can lead to a nonproductive cycle of more stress and depression, leaving you less able to meet daily challenges. And, if you become physically run down, your immune system becomes less resistant to infection and illness. In this chapter, we will provide some tools to help you decipher the causes of your fatigue and strategies for managing it. Although some fatigue may be unavoidable, you can eliminate certain sources and triggers of fatigue by being a good self-manager. By setting priorities, making smart choices and conserving your strength, you will still be able to do most of what is important to you.

Pinpointing Causes of Your Fatigue

Your fatigue may be caused by physical, emotional and environmental factors. The box on page 210 provides a list of some of the more common physical and emotional causes of fatigue, and lists some actions that you can take to address them.

Identifying the Causes of Your Fatigue

Physical Causes

Are you experiencing a flare of rheumatoid arthritis? The process of inflammation can make you feel tired all over.
Action: Discuss a possible change in your treatment plan, such as increasing dosages of medication to control the flare.

Are you overdoing activities or pushing yourself too hard? Fatigue can be a signal that you are doing too much.
Action: Cut down on the number of tasks you do each day. Learn to alternate periods of activity and breaks.

Have you been doing very little? Too much inactivity leads to muscle deconditioning and can actually make you feel worse.
Action: Incorporate more physical activity into your daily routine (see Chapter 14). A therapist can show you safe and gentle exercises that won't harm your joints.

Are you taking any new medications? Fatigue can be a side effect of some.
Action: Talk to your doctor or pharmacist about your concerns. It may be possible to switch medications or take them at different times during the day.

Do you awaken feeling rested? If not, you may have insomnia caused by pain.
Action: Your doctor or pharmacist may suggest medications that can ease your pain or help you sleep. Also see tips on getting a good night's sleep in this chapter.

In addition to these, environmental factors such as high noise levels, temperature variations, and even daily hassles such as dealing with traffic and waiting in line can make you feel tired.

Keeping a Fatigue Diary

One way to help you discover the causes of your fatigue is to keep a fatigue diary similar to the one shown here. In it, you can note the times of the day or week when you feel fatigue and also what seems to trigger the feeling. Although it may seem like a lot of work, sometimes you may see an obvious solution to the problem that you might otherwise miss. For instance, you may blame overactivity when you feel tired, but by reviewing your diary you may

Is your fatigue accompanied by all-over muscle pain or tenderness? If so, you may have fibromyalgia in addition to your arthritis.

Action: Describe your symptoms to your doctor. He or she may prescribe an additional medication, or provide exercise or relaxation tips.

Emotional Causes

Are you experiencing more stress than usual? Your body's response to stress uses up energy, particularly if the stress is continuous.

Action: Track your stress using a diary, as discussed in Chapter 18. Prioritize your tasks to conserve energy.

Have you been worrying more lately? It's natural to have worries and concerns, particularly when you have a chronic disease. However, worry drains energy and can become a compulsive habit.

Action: Try using relaxation techniques or sharing your concerns with your spouse or a friend. Write down your worries and then try to find solutions.

Do you feel depressed? People who have clinical depression often experience fatigue.

Action: Seek professional help if you think you may have symptoms of depression. Also, read Chapter 14 for information on dealing with depression.

see that your fatigue is actually a sign of increased disease activity that calls for a change in your treatment plan. You may wish to discuss this with your doctor.

What Your Doctor Can Do

When fatigue is due to inflammation, it is often more easily corrected than when it is due to stress. The inflammatory cytokines (protein molecules) that are released in rheumatoid arthritis are the same chemicals that are released when you have a severe cold or flu. Although in rheumatoid arthritis they are not fighting to protect your body from disease, they can still leave you feeling weak and tired. Your doctor can improve this type of fatigue by prescribing higher doses of your drugs or another drug to be used alone or in combination to control the body's inflammatory process. Once inflammation is under control, fatigue usually lessens.

It is also important to consider other potential sources of fatigue that your doctor can reverse. One possibility is anemia, which occurs when the body has too few red blood cells to transport oxygen effectively.

A Sample Fatigue Diary

CAUSE OF FATIGUE	POSSIBLE SOLUTIONS
10 a.m. – Parent-teacher conference at school	*Cancel other appointments that day; plan for afternoon rest time*

One type of anemia, also called "the anemia of chronic disease," is often seen in people with rheumatoid arthritis. Effective treatment of arthritis usually resolves this type of anemia. Another cause of anemia is blood loss from stomach ulcers, which may require iron replacement and other treatments.

Another consideration is the medications themselves. Fatigue is a side effect of many medications, most frequently drugs for other conditions such as hypertension (high blood pressure) or depression. Ask your doctor if any medications you are taking cause fatigue, and whether any adjustments can be made to improve the situation.

Fibromyalgia (see Chapter 5) is also common in people with rheumatoid arthritis, and may cause fatigue.

If you have a second chronic condition (that is, a medical condition in addition to rheumatoid arthritis), your level of fatigue may be even higher. For instance, people with thyroid disease or lung problems often feel fatigued for reasons other than inflammation. If you and your doctor address these additional problems, your level of energy should increase.

Sometimes fatigue can be aggravated by not being able to get a good night's sleep. Although we will discuss some ways

that you can improve your sleep habits, another option is the use of sleeping pills. Some people with rheumatoid arthritis have an excellent experience with sleeping pills, but others find pills don't work well. You can work with your doctor to determine the best approach and which sleeping pills might work best for you.

What You Can Do

The most effective approach you can take when dealing with your fatigue is to be aware that fatigue is a part of rheumatoid arthritis, and that you might have to adapt your schedule to the fatigue, rather than fighting it. Don't look at your fatigue as a sign of personal weakness or try to deny it. It is simply one more symptom of your arthritis that you can learn to handle.

For example, many people with rheumatoid arthritis adjust their daily schedule, starting their day one or two hours later than they once did. This makes it easier to deal with morning stiffness and may also enable you to sleep longer. Ultimately, the result is less fatigue and a more productive day. Other people may take a rest or nap in the afternoon, which then allows them to continue their daily activities without collapsing from exhaustion at the end of the day.

214

"When I was 10 years old, my mother was diagnosed with rheumatoid arthritis in an era when not much was known about the disease, and there were no support groups. At 31, I was also diagnosed with rheumatoid arthritis. I was devastated, but I quickly learned the value of the Arthritis Foundation and its wealth of guidance and educational materials.

"The first step was to choose a physician, one I had a good rapport with. I knew the doctor would be a major part of my life – and my friend. I have learned a lot of emotional coping and self-management skills from others. Hopefully, sharing these skills will help someone else, like the sharing other people have done with me over the years. The skills are:

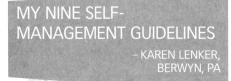

MY NINE SELF-
MANAGEMENT GUIDELINES

– KAREN LENKER,
BERWYN, PA

1. Before my feet hit the ground in the morning, I think of 10 things to be grateful for.

2. Exercise in the morning, either walking, riding a stationary bike, or doing exercises or water aerobics at the YMCA.

3. Take time dressing and grooming. Nice soap, cologne, attention to jewelry, or a scarf can perk you up. Most major stores have personal shoppers, and this service can save you lots of energy.

4. Schedule ahead so your days aren't so busy. Include time for rest.

5. Make lists to save time. I always keep a small notepad with me. Doctor's appointments are more productive when I take a list of subjects to be addressed.

6. Educate family and friends about your arthritis by talking with them or offering them printed material from the Arthritis Foundation.

7. Ask for help ahead of an event, so others can put you in their schedules. Sometimes I give a family member a written list to eliminate constant asking.

8. Have fun. Church, hobbies, movies and reading will keep you connected with other people. Support groups are invaluable.

9. Do something for someone else. Help someone with an errand, visit or listening ear. Correspond with an old friend or relative. Volunteer."

Using a fatigue diary can help you determine when you feel most tired, and help you adjust your schedule accordingly. Is it right after a heavy lunch? Or do you get sleepy after working at the computer all morning? Try varying your tasks and taking brief breaks to stretch and move around. If you are able, plan to take a walk during your lunch hour a few days a week. Avoid eating heavy meals; instead, opt for a light lunch, perhaps with a healthy morning and afternoon snack thrown in.

Rest is crucial. But recognizing that doing too little can often lead to deconditioning is also important – which in turn makes you feel more fatigued. Moderate exercise keeps your muscles and joints in condition, and has the added benefit of helping you sleep better at night. The conventional wisdom that you get energy by using it is true.

Understanding Your Body's Rhythms

Recent research has shown that people have natural tendencies to be most awake at certain hours and most rested at others. These patterns are referred to as your body's circadian rhythms. Most people seem to be "morning people" and have their most alert hours in the morning, tend to go to sleep by 9:00 to 11:00 p.m.,

sleep for seven to eight hours, and awaken between 6:00 and 7:00 a.m. However, some people are "night people" who find it difficult to get up in the morning and feel tired all day if they are forced to get up before restful sleep can occur.

For years, scientists believed that people could change their body's natural rhythms, but new findings suggest these adjustments are more complex than first thought. A night person who has to arise before 6:00 a.m. may often feel fatigued all day, unless a nap is possible. Study your own body's natural rhythms, and you may be able to determine the best time to go to sleep and wake up. Of course, planning your daily schedule completely is impossible, but the more you can be in harmony with your natural rhythms, the less likely you will suffer from a high level of fatigue.

Getting a Good Night's Sleep

A lack of restful sleep is a problem shared by many Americans – and caused by different factors: stress; depression; caffeine, alcohol or drugs; not allowing enough time for sleep; and pain. When you have rheumatoid arthritis, pain may keep you from falling asleep easily, or it may awaken you during the night. Research has shown that some people with rheumatoid

Checklist for Getting the Sleep You Need

Establish Regular Sleep Patterns

- Try to go to bed and get up at the same time each day.

- Avoid taking naps too close to bedtime.

- Take a warm- to-hot bath within two hours of bedtime.

- A warm non-caffeinated drink may help you relax.

Create a Restful Environment

- Make sure your bedroom is dark, quiet and comfortable.

- Avoid bright light if you have to get up during the sleep period.

- Keep your clock turned away from you.

Exercise

- Exercise regularly each day.

- Avoid vigorous exercise or activity for at least two hours prior to bedtime.

Be Aware of Drug Effects

- Give up smoking, or avoid smoking several hours before bedtime.

- Limit use of alcoholic beverages.

- Cut back or discontinue drinking caffeinated beverages.

- Use prescribed sleep medication only as directed.

Other Considerations

- Avoid large meals two to three hours before bedtime.

- Menopause and aging may cause changes to your established sleep patterns.

- If pain keeps you from sleeping, discuss medication options with your doctor.

Reprinted from *Clinical Care in the Rheumatic Diseases*. Used with permission of the American College of Rheumatology.

arthritis experience light, easily disrupted sleep with many mid-sleep awakenings. This leads to higher levels of fatigue.

There are several stages of sleep. During the night, your brain moves between these stages in cycles, and the types of electrical brain waves generated vary from stage to stage. To feel rested, your brain requires what is called "delta sleep," named after the brain waves that occur in the third and fourth stages of sleep. REM (short for rapid eye movement) sleep is also important. It's the stage of sleep when dreaming occurs, and without it, you will feel tired.

Aging and menopause cause changes in sleep patterns. As people age, the amount and quality of sleep they get varies. Older individuals tend to spend less time in deep (restorative) sleep and to sleep for shorter periods. Menopause, which usually occurs in the late 40s through early 50s, can also cause sleep disturbances such as hot flashes and frequent awakenings. Hormone replacement therapy may help alleviate these symptoms.

So, how can you get the sleep you need? Review the checklist on this page for some helpful suggestions, but be aware that it may take time to change your ingrained patterns. If you feel anxious about getting to sleep, consider adding relaxation exercises to your nighttime routine as well.

Prioritizing Your Time and Energy

There may be times when you feel more fatigued than others, and you will have to deal with limitations to your energy. Think of your energy as a resource that you have to conserve for your most important activities. This may involve saying no to lower priority activities that take up too much of your energy.

Of course, saying no is not always easy, but it helps you stay focused on the priorities in your life, such as earning a living or spending time with your children. When you're feeling fatigued, opting out of an activity may allow you to get the rest you need. Saying no to one activity may allow you to say yes to something more important to you. Chapter 20 provides additional ideas about prioritizing your activities and conserving your energy.

Ask for Help, Even If It's Difficult

Successful managers are people who have learned that they cannot do everything themselves. Borrowing from their techniques, you can learn to delegate tasks that will help you manage your activities. Asking for help may be difficult at first. Because the effects of rheumatoid arthritis are not always visible to the outside observer, you may be afraid that co-workers and acquaintances will perceive you as lazy.

You may feel embarrassed to ask for help, especially if you've always viewed yourself as a high achiever. The following suggestions can make it easier to request help.

- **Ask for specific help.** For example, if you ask someone to take you shopping for one hour every other Tuesday morning, you are letting them know precisely the help you need. Also, you show others that you understand their time is valuable.

- **Develop a pool of helpers.** Spreading out the load of tasks keeps the burden from falling on any one person. Keep a list of friends and family and the tasks they're willing to help with.

- **Consider bartering or trading services.** If you dislike asking for help, perhaps you can provide a service in return. For instance, offer to watch your friend's children one afternoon a week at your house, if she will run some errands for you.

PART FIVE

Mastering Emotional Challenges

Chapter 18

Mind Power:
Getting Mentally Tough

Can you really affect your rheumatoid arthritis – positively or negatively – by having a certain outlook? The answer is yes. The major question is how much – and that probably differs greatly from person to person (like everything else with rheumatoid arthritis).

Findings over the last few years indicate that how you react to the stresses and challenges of living with a chronic disease may influence the course of the disease. Equally important, your outlook may influence your long-term ability to keep doing the daily activities that keep you independent and help make your life meaningful.

You can explore different strategies to help you deal with your arthritis. This chapter presents some ideas about how the mind-body connection works, and why it affects your arthritis. It also looks at some of the techniques shown to be effective self-management tools.

The Mind-Body Connection

In the past, doctors believed in a "rheumatoid arthritis personality." Some researchers had a theory that rheumatoid arthritis could be considered a psychosomatic disease – meaning that "mental" processes led to physical disease.

As we now know, this idea was an oversimplification of a complicated situation. There is no such thing as a rheumatoid arthritis personality; all types of people get rheumatoid arthritis, and the disease affects people in different ways. However, there was a germ of truth in the idea. It does appear that the mind plays some role in the disease process in rheumatoid arthritis – and most diseases.

For instance, a person's reaction to stressful events probably has an effect on flares of rheumatoid arthritis in some, if not most, people. Continued stress appears to make it harder to control disease. People with optimistic outlooks and feelings of being in control tend to do better long-term than those with less positive feelings about their rheumatoid arthritis. The concept of being in control is known as *self-efficacy*, and its opposite as *helplessness*. We'll discuss the cornerstones of positive mental strategies in this chapter.

Why Self-Efficacy Can Help

As you know, rheumatoid arthritis is a chronic, painful condition that can cause stress, frustration and depression. These in turn make pain worse. The cycle of pain is vicious, but it can be halted or reduced through treatment, and by learning to deal with pain in positive, constructive ways.

Some people who have rheumatoid arthritis may believe their situation is uncontrollable and no effective solutions can help them, a situation known as helplessness.

A Pioneer Course Still Going Strong

The Arthritis Foundation Self-Help Program was developed in 1979 by Stanford University researchers Kate Lorig, RN, DrPH, and James Fries, MD. It sprang from a groundbreaking idea: to provide people with arthritis with information about the disease and the skills to help them regain control of their lives. "The point of the course," explains Dr. Lorig, "is to help people have more confidence about managing their symptoms and live a better life with the disease." Leaders trained and certified by the Arthritis Foundation teach the classes.

To help people control their arthritis, the six-week program emphasizes self-efficacy skills, along with cognitive pain management, effective communication between doctors and patients, and aerobic exercises. In one research study, individuals who attended the program reduced their pain by 20 percent and visits to physicians by 40 percent. The success of the course has spurred the development of other programs that also help people cope with chronic pain and learn self-efficacy techniques.

To locate an Arthritis Foundation Self-Help Program near you, contact the Arthritis Foundation by telephone at 800-568-4045, or online at www.arthritis.org. Ask for the office of the Arthritis Foundation chapter nearest you. The chapter staff will be able to guide you to resources in your area.

The feelings may result in anxiety, depression and fear of the future. People may lose interest in daily living and in learning new skills that could help them manage pain and stress.

Self-efficacy, which refers to a person's feeling that she or he can master a specific situation, can help people with rheumatoid arthritis cope better with their disease than those who feel helpless in the face of constantly fluctuating symptoms.

Self-efficacy is specific to situations, rather than an overall approach to coping. Actually, a layman's term for self-efficacy is confidence. For instance, a person who has rheumatoid arthritis but also has self-efficacy may believe she can walk around the block, and eventually even walk a mile or two (depending on her doctor's advice). But that doesn't mean she has to believe she can climb Mount Everest.

The good news is that helplessness may be overcome and self-efficacy skills learned. When researchers discovered the importance of optimism and self-efficacy, they began to develop programs and courses to help people with arthritis learn these skills. One of the first programs – and still one of the most successful – is the Arthritis Foundation Self-Help Program, offered through the Arthritis Foundation (see box on the previous page). During the course, participants learn and practice self-efficacy skills that help them manage their disease.

Coping with Stress

Having rheumatoid arthritis increases physical and emotional challenges. You may feel fear, anger and frustration about your pain or physical limitations. These emotions are normal and are part of the process your body goes through to make sense of the new situation in your life. Some people are able to experience these emotions and move on, but many others who have rheumatoid arthritis find it difficult to deal with the ongoing stresses of chronic disease. Finding ways to do that should be a component of your self-management plan.

What Is Stress?

Stress refers to the body's physical, mental and chemical reactions to frightening, exciting, dangerous or irritating circumstances. This can be anything from getting the children to school on time to avoiding a crash on the freeway. Every day we face hundreds of stresses – some big, some small – that we have to respond to.

When we face stress, our bodies respond by releasing adrenaline, cortisol

Putting Stress in Perspective

You can learn to take a more objective look at the stresses and stress-causing patterns in your life by asking yourself these questions:

- Does this situation present a threat (harm), or a challenge (opportunity)?

- Are there other ways to look at this situation?

- What is at stake?

- What are you saying to yourself right now? Is it productive?

- What are you afraid will occur?

- What evidence do you have that this will happen?

- Is there evidence that contradicts this conclusion?

- What changes can you make?

- What coping resources are available to you?

and other hormones into the bloodstream. The hormones increase heart rate, blood pressure and muscle tension, and induce the "fight or flight response." This response works fine most of the time. In fact, it can be beneficial, particularly during emergencies or in high-pressure situations. However, after a stressful situation is resolved, the body's pace needs to return to normal.

Unfortunately, stress levels in our modern society are high. You probably experience daily stress on the job, in traffic or because of your health. If you are unable to release tension between stressful situations, your body may start to respond to every pressure as an emergency. Think of your body as a car: It's unhealthy to race your engine constantly. You need to shift into neutral to save wear and tear on your engine.

When the stress response continues for an extended period, it can wear you down. You may find yourself reaching overload and notice that you are accident-prone or that you are making more mistakes than usual – signs that you need to relieve some of the stress in your life.

Managing Stress

By using methods that have been developed by clinicians and people with arthritis, and tested by researchers, you can improve your own stress-management skills. The first step is to identify what is causing stress in your life (these factors are called stressors). Second, you should try to eliminate as many stressors as possible. The third step is to develop effective coping mechanisms to help you counteract the stresses that you cannot eliminate. Some coping mechanisms that can help you manage stress include progressive muscle relaxation, guided imagery, deep breathing techniques and active problem solving.

Step one: *Identifying stressors.* Before you can change or manage your stress, you must become aware of what's causing it. Identifying your stressors is a process of personal discovery. Of course, universal stresses – such as moving, changing jobs or having a baby – affect every person's life. But in your daily life, other stressors are highly individual. What triggers stress for you may not necessarily bother someone else.

One way to discover what causes you stress is to keep a stress diary. The sample diary shown here is a way to note the things that cause you to feel "stressed

out." Review your entries at the end of each week to see if there is a pattern of stress-related events. Some people find that this step alone can be empowering. Indeed, extensive research indicates that the simple act of writing down difficulties can lead to better outcomes.

The physical signs of stress can also provide clues to note in your stress diary. These include tiredness/exhaustion, tense muscles, upset stomach, insomnia, cold sweaty hands, changes in appetite, teeth grinding, jaw clenching, and general body complaints such as weakness, dizziness, headache or muscle pain. Many of these physical symptoms of stress are also symptoms of arthritis. For example, fatigue, weakness and muscle pain are common in rheumatoid arthritis, especially during a flare. So, sometimes it may be difficult to tell whether your symptoms are caused by stress or by disease; often it's both.

Your stress diary might also include emotional symptoms. These can range from mild irritability to feelings of depression. Anxiety, nervousness and agitation are also common signs of stress. Be as specific as possible, so that you can target the most troublesome areas for you.

Step two: *Eliminate the negative.* Now comes the challenging part: trying to weed out negative pressures in your life. Obviously, not all negative stressors can be eliminated, and sometimes just thinking about changes in your life is stressful. For instance, you may feel obligated to honor many family and volunteer duties. It may seem easier to continue doing them than to back out. Others may pressure you not to change. But you need to realize that saying no to a few of these obligations may enable you to feel less stressed and have more energy for the things you really must or want to do.

Review your stress diary. Are there predictable times during the day or week when you feel particularly hassled? For example, being stuck in rush-hour traffic may disrupt your equilibrium and deplete the energy you need to see you through the day. Brainstorm for options that could make your commute easier. Can you leave for work earlier? Can you carpool or take public transportation? Would listening to your favorite classical music make you feel more relaxed? Now try taking each problem you've identified and see if you can figure out ways to reduce the stress associated with each.

Carrying out this step may be especially difficult for people who pride themselves on their competency and efficiency. But no one is immune to stressful stimuli.

Adjust your mindset by remembering that the more stress you eliminate, the more productively you will handle tasks you must do. If you can take a step back and become more objective about your situation, evaluating and dealing with stress will be easier.

Step three: *Develop effective coping mechanisms.* A positive attitude can contribute to relieving the cycle of stress in your life. Of course, simply looking on the sunny side cannot make a serious problem go away. But by cultivating flexibility and learning how to deal with change, you will feel less stress and be able to deal with problems more effectively.

There are many ways to counteract stress. For example, if you find yourself dwelling on your problems, you can learn to refocus your attention on solving them and on positive things you enjoy. Thinking about something you like can help you relax and become less stressed. Also, humor is a wonderful way to relieve stress. Schedule time for play, and become involved in activities that make you laugh.

Another key is to develop and use support systems. Sharing your thoughts with family, friends, clergy or other good listeners can help you view your problems in a constructive way. A support group of people who have arthritis may provide a valuable source of both listeners and information on dealing with stress.

When you feel that stress is about to overwhelm you, develop a "safety valve" procedure to let off steam. This could involve writing down your feelings in a journal, taking some time to calm down in a quiet setting, or exercising vigorously (but safely). Above all, try to keep a balance between your work, family and recreation. Don't feel that you have to eliminate all your fun activities to conserve your energy for work and/or family obligations. That will increase your stress and your resentment. Many people with rheumatoid arthritis find that staying busy

and concentrating on something other than arthritis boosts their sense of well-being and helps sustain their spirits during times of pain or diminished activity.

Another positive way to handle stress is to take good care of your body. Make every effort to eat a balanced diet, exercise, and get enough rest and sleep. Learn to listen to your body for physical signs of stress: If your head aches or your heart is beating fast during everyday situations – when you're driving or cooking dinner, for example – you may be pushing too hard.

Learning to Relax

The ability to relax can help you relieve symptoms of stress, including tight muscles, fast

Sample Stress Diary

DATE	CAUSE OF STRESS	TIME	PHYSICAL SYMPTOMS	EMOTIONAL SYMPTOMS
4/18	getting kids off to school	7 a.m.	fast heartbeat, tightness of neck	feel rushed, disorganized
4/18	stuck in traffic	8:30 a.m.	headache, heart beating faster, legs aching	frustrated, angry at being late
4/18	meeting presentation	10 a.m.	fast heartbeat, dry throat, clammy palms	anxious, nervous

and shallow breathing, fast heart rate, and high blood pressure. In addition, feeling relaxed helps you have a sense of well-being and control, which contributes to your ability to cope with stress. Learning relaxation techniques is not easy, especially if you are in pain.

If you would like to try some simple imagery and relaxation exercises, several

Stress Diary

Keep a diary or chart if you can and record the causes of your stress as well as physical or emotional symptoms you experience. Keeping a stress diary can help you learn what causes your stress and how you can avoid it. Photocopy this chart or create your own version.

DATE	CAUSE OF STRESS	TIME	PHYSICAL SYMPTOMS	EMOTIONAL SYMPTOMS

are listed at the end of this chapter. Again, remember that these take practice. Don't expect immediate results. It may be several weeks before you reap benefits from some techniques.

Activity: Deep Breathing

Deep breathing is a basic technique that is a part of almost all relaxation exercises and a key to unwinding. Here are the steps:

1. Get as comfortable as you can. Loosen any tight clothing, take off restricting jewelry, and uncross your legs and arms. Close your eyes.

2. Place your hands firmly but comfortably on your stomach. This will help you feel when you are breathing properly. When you breathe correctly, your stomach expands t as you breathe in and contracts when you breathe out. (Many people breathe "backward" – they tighten their stomachs when they breathe in and relax their stomachs when they breathe out. If you're a "backwards breather," take a minute to coordinate your movements and breath.)

3. Inhale slowly and deeply through your nose to a count of three. Feel your stomach push against your hands? Let it expand as much as possible as you fill your lungs with air.

4. When your lungs are full, purse your lips (as if you were going to whistle) and exhale slowly through your mouth for a count of six. (Pursing your lips allows you to control how slowly you exhale.) Feel your stomach shrink away from your hands.

5. When your lungs feel empty, close your mouth and begin the inhale-exhale cycle again. Repeat the cycle three or four times at each session.

6. Whenever you're ready, slowly open your eyes and stretch.

Tip: Breathing deeply can make you feel light-headed or dizzy, especially when you are tired or hungry. At first, practice deep breathing while you are sitting or lying down. Once you get the hang of it, deep breathing can be done anytime, anyplace.

Activity: Relaxation to Control Pain
Beginning Part
(excerpted from "Imaginative Progressive Relaxation" technique):

First, take some time to make sure that you are in a comfortable position. Make a quick check from head to toe to determine whether your whole body is supported. Adjust any parts that feel uncomfortable. Try not to have legs or arms crossed, but do what is comfortable for you.

Now, close your eyes. Become aware of your breathing. Feel the movement of your body as you breathe in and out. Breathe in slowly and exhale. On your next breath, focus on the image of breathing in good, clean air , exhaling all your tensions with your breath out. Allow your breathing rhythm to slow down. Each time you breathe out notice the tension you release.

Middle Part:

Option 1: *"Pain Drain"* Note where you experience pain or tension. Imagine that the pain or tension is turning into a liquid substance. The heavy liquid flows through your body and out through your fingers and toes. Allow the pain to drain from your body in a steady flow. Now, imagine that the water from a gentle rain flows over your head, further dissolving the pain into a liquid that drains away. Enjoy the sense of comfort and well-being that follows.

Option 2: *"Disappearing Pain"* Notice any tension or pain that you are experiencing. Imagine that the pain takes the form of an object or several objects – fruit, pebbles, crystals, or anything else that comes to mind. Pick each piece of pain, one at a time, and place it in a magic box.

As you drop each piece into the box, it dissolves into nothingness. Look within your body to see if pieces remain. Imagine that your body is lighter and

allow yourself to experience comfort and a sense of well-being. Enjoy this feeling of tranquility and repose.

Option 3: *"Healing Potion"* Imagine you are in a drugstore stocked with bottles and jars of exotic potions. Each potion has a magical quality. Some are pure, white light, others are lotions, balms and creams, and still others contain healing vibrations. As you survey the potions, choose one that appeals to you. It may even have your name on the container. Open the container and cover your body with the magical potion. As you apply it, let pain or tension melt away, leaving you with a feeling of comfort and well-being. Imagine that you place the container in a special spot and that it continually renews its contents for future use.

Option 4: *"Leaving Pain Behind"* Imagine that you are dreaming. Although your body stays in the same position, imagine that you are gently leaving it. As you leave your body, notice that you have also left your tension and pain behind. Pick a special spot to visit, one that brings pleasure and a feeling of well-being. Notice how your now dreamlike body feels as you visit this special place. Linger here and when you feel ready, return to the body you left behind. When you open your eyes, retain the freedom from tension and pain, and continue to experience a sense of comfort and well-being.

End Part:

Whenever you are ready, slowly stretch and open your eyes.

Adapted from The ROM Dance, a range-of-motion and relaxation program, Diane Harlowe and Patricia Yu, 1992. Published by St. Mary's Hospital Medical Center, Madison, WI. Materials available from The ROM Dance, 408 S. Baldwin Street, Madison, WI 53703. 800/488-4940. www.taichihealth.com

Activity: Guided-Imagery Smorgasbord

Think of guided imagery as a daydream with a tour guide. By diverting your attention from stress, guided imagery takes your mind on a mini-vacation. Use your imagination to transport yourself to a more peaceful place. For some people the most relaxing place is the seashore, for others the mountains. Pick your mind's ideal vacation spot and go there. The following exercise teaches you how to focus on relaxing in your choice of desirable, stress-free locations. Have a friend read the exercise to you – or record it yourself and play it back as you imagine.

Beginning ritual:

Get as comfortable as you can, feet slightly apart, arms resting at your sides. Now close your eyes. Take a slow deep breath through your nose and slowly exhale through your mouth. Again, take a deep breath and slowly exhale. Continue to breathe slowly and deeply. Notice yourself getting more and more relaxed. Let all your tension melt away.

Middle part:

Option 1: *"Sea"* Your body is heavy, at ease and warm. Listen to your heart beating steadily and regularly. As you listen to your heart, you feel its beat in your whole body. It feels as though you are on a boat on a quiet calm sea with the water lapping against the sides.

You're inhaling and exhaling like the waves gently rocking you. The rocking continues in your mind, and as you rock, the negative emotions drop out of you, one after the other – frustration, sorrow, depression, heartache, worries, resentment. You feel serene and content. You feel so wonderful you'd like the whole world to enjoy the feeling with you, and out of the depths of your heart rises a great lightness. You feel it flow in a steady stream through your whole body, and all the time you feel lighter and lighter.

Adapted from the Arthritis Movement Workshop Leader's Manual, Arthritis Foundation, Arizona Chapter.

Option 2: *"Pine Forest"* Imagine in as much detail as possible that you are sitting comfortably in a chair or hammock in the middle of a beautiful pine forest. Enjoy the fresh, cool, clean, fragrant air. What a pleasure it is to breathe. Imagine the gentle, cool breeze as it touches your skin.

You are sitting comfortably, feeling peaceful and calm. As you look around, you are impressed by the beauty of the tall pine trees with their rich brown bark and graceful feathery green branches. You notice the pinecones on the branches. You watch the leaves of the aspen trees dancing in the wind. The ground interests you with its rich brown dirt covered with pine needles and leaves and its robust, earthy aroma.

You hear birds calling and a woodpecker at work in the distance. You notice a small clearing in the forest. The clearing is covered with green grass and beautiful wildflowers of all types and colors. You see butterflies around the flowers. You are at peace in your pine forest, sitting comfortably, feeling relaxed and calm appreciating the wonders of nature and of being alive.

Adapted from the Multiple Sclerosis Self-Help Course Leader's Guide by Katalina McGlone, 1984.

Option 3: *"Ocean Beach"* Imagine that you are at the ocean. You are sitting comfortably on the beach under the shade of a large beach umbrella. Feel the warm sand under you…and the warm, comfortable air around you, the refreshing, soft breeze blowing through your hair. Feel the warm moisture in the air upon your face Notice the smell of the ocean. Imagine how beautiful, brilliantly blue the sky is

You're sitting on the beach feeling calm, peaceful, relaxed, comfortable. You are watching the waves as they grow and break, mesmerized as they go in and out from the shore. You can hear the thundering of the waves, the cries of the seagulls. Notice how peaceful you feel sitting on the beach feeling in harmony with nature.

Adapted from the Systemic Lupus Erythematosus Self-Help Course Leader's Manual – Katalina McGlone, 1984.

Option 4: *"Floating in Space"* Imagine you are standing on a mat in front of an elevator. The doors open, you step in and watch the numbers slowly change: 1, 2, 3, 4, 5, 6, 7, 8, 9, 10. The doors open, and you step out into deep, dark outer space. Feel yourself floating weightlessly, drifting, light. See the velvety blue of space around you. Look at the earth, small and green. Imagine stars and planets moving past you. Imagine yourself moving towards a space of diffuse white light, as bright and ethereal as a distant star. As you approach this light, it increases in size until you feel yourself surrounded by its glow. You feel that you are bathed in feelings of tranquility and well-being.

If disturbing thoughts or feelings enter your mind, allow them to pass by you, just as you imagine planets and stars passing. Let these thoughts and feelings fade, leaving them behind like comets disappearing over the horizon.

Personally Speaking STORIES FROM REAL PEOPLE

"I wonder if a single person exists out there who has some golden years to her credit and been diagnosed with rheumatoid arthritis, who hasn't experienced this:

"I go into the bathroom housing the same facilities I've been using for umpteen years, and all of a sudden they aren't facilities anymore – they're obstacles. The appliance that set the most unique trap for me is the toilet seat, in our household referred to as the 'johnny seat.'

VANITY WORKS FOR ME
– BETTY MOORE, LUKEVILLE, AZ

"Sitting down isn't too much of a problem, even though at times, my knees don't want to bend as easily as they used to, and I land with a thud. But the process of getting up is tough, beginning what I term the 'johnny rock.' Getting up off that booby trap has turned me into a contortionist, with my arthritis gnawing at my joints. My mind says, 'OK, I'm ready to get up.' Every fiber in my body tells me to stand up. But there I sit. I brace my hands so they can help me force myself up and off. That's when the rocking begins. I rock back thinking, 'This time I will push myself up and off this seat.' But I seem to have a magnet sewn onto my bottom, and the johnny seat is made of steel.

"I feel defeated, and then the ultimate motivation possesses of me. If I can't get off this seat, I will have to call for help from my husband. An extra surge of adrenaline flows through my veins, I push with my hands and shoulders, and no matter the pain, zap! I'm standing. Vanity – no doubt about it – works for me."

Enjoy the peaceful feelings of this place. Slowly float out of the white light, imagining that it has filled your body and you are carrying it with you. Then float back past the stars and planets through the blue space to the elevator. Step back in, see the doors close, watch the numbers change: 10, 9, 8, 7, 6, 5, 4, 3, 2, 1. The doors open and you feel your body on the mat.

Adapted from the Arthritis Movement Workshop Leader's Manual, Arthritis Foundation, Arizona Chapter.

Option 5: *"Memory and Fantasy"* In this relaxation exercise, remember a past experience – or create a new one – with your imagination.

Imagine yourself in an environment where you feel secure, comfortable and relaxed. This can be a place you remember, a fantasy you are creating or a mixture of memory and imagination. Experience whatever comes to you. Sometimes the environment will change during the exercise, and sometimes it will remain the same.

Place yourself in this environment and note how you are positioned: standing, sitting, or lying down. In this relaxed environment, look around you. Take in the panorama of colors, forms and textures. If you are outside or can see outside, note the season, time of day or night, and the weather. Look all around

you – in front, behind both sides, above and below you. Look at the sky or ceiling, the ground or floor, in the distance and up close. Are there other people here? Take in all you wish to see. What sounds come to you? Listen for sounds in the distance, up close, all around you. Where do the sounds come from?

In this comfortable environment, is there anything that you can smell? If something to drink or eat presents itself, savor it and note its texture in your mouth. Is there anything or anybody you are touching? How does it feel?

How does the environment around you feel physically? Warm or cool? Damp or dry? Do you feel movement in the air? How does it feel emotionally? How do you feel inside in this environment?

Once again, take in the sights around you. They may have changed. Note the sounds, smells, tastes, and sights. Focus on emotional feelings, the feelings inside you.

Adapted from The ROM Dance, a range-of-motion and relaxation program, Diane Harlowe and Patricia Yu, 1992. Materials available from The ROM Dance, 408 S. Baldwin Street, Madison, WI 53703. 800/488-4940. www.taichihealth.com

Option 6: *"Water Fantasy"* Imagine that you are immersed in water, perhaps in your bathtub, in a lake, swimming pool, or even a whirlpool bath. Imagine that the water is the perfect temperature, just warm enough so that every muscle in your body feels as supple and flowing as the very water itself. Experience the water flowing around and coming into contact with each part of you. As it does this, it melts away deeper levels of tension, leaving your whole body feeling cleansed and drained of all tension.

Let yourself stay in the water for a while, letting go of deeper and deeper levels of tension and allowing yourself to feel more and more relaxed.

Adapted from The ROM Dance.

End Part:

(Silence)…You may go back to this place whenever you want, simply by sitting quietly and remembering this place in as much detail as possible. Whenever you are ready, move your fingers, wiggle your toes, and come back to this world feeling refreshed and invigorated.

Build up your resistance to stress. Stress can have a negative effect on your body. Taking good care of your body can help you build up resistance to stress. Ways to do that include:

- eating a balanced diet
- exercising
- avoiding drugs and alcohol
- getting enough rest and sleep
- saving energy by pacing your activities
- accentuating the positive.

Incorporate the relaxation techniques you've learned in this chapter into your daily life and you'll reap rewards. Managing your stress – whether or not you have rheumatoid arthritis – can lessen pain and increase good living.

Chapter 19

Losses and Gains:
Getting Past Grief and Depression

Chronic illness may change your life in so many ways that you'll sometimes wonder if you're the same person. It's not surprising that after the initial relief of diagnosis, when you have a name for your problem at last, grief sets in. Yet this pervasive feeling of loss catches many people with rheumatoid arthritis by surprise.

What Is Grief?

Grief is a natural response to loss. Usually, we associate grief with death or divorce. Feelings of grief over the diagnosis of a chronic illness are not discussed very often, but chronic illness, too, involves loss.

For people with rheumatoid arthritis, the losses are physical, social and personal. Mourning these losses is not only natural, but necessary as part of a healing process that allows you to accept the changes your disease has brought.

Giving yourself permission to grieve for your old life will help you reach acceptance sooner and put you on the path to building a new life. Your spouse and family members also may need to grieve about the changes in your health. Allow them to do it in their own way and time.

If You Experience Depression

Anyone who develops an illness – particularly a chronic illness such as rheumatoid arthritis – may experience psychological distress. This may manifest itself as feelings of depression and helplessness. Not everyone experiences these feelings, but if you do recognizing them is important, the first step to finding ways to deal with the distress.

Depression

Most people occasionally feels "down" or "blue," and they may refer to the feelings as "being depressed." Clinical depression,

Possible Grief Responses

- **Shock and denial: "No! It can't be true!"** Denial is a protective buffer, allowing you to replace anxious thoughts with more hopeful ones. Denial buys time for you to mobilize other coping techniques and face your losses at a manageable pace. This stage is usually temporary, but if you can't accept your diagnosis, you won't be able to fight your condition.

- **Bargaining: "Let's make a deal.** "You may find yourself making secret promises, for example, "I'll become a better person" if fate or a higher power sends a cure. Or you may begin an endless cycle of seeking other medical opinions and trying unproven remedies. This process is yet another "time-buying" stage before acceptance.

- **Anger: "Why me?"** Anger, rage, envy and resentment are all common responses to bad news like a diagnosis of RA. You may express your anger by criticizing your doctor, family or friends. You may put off necessary chores or treatments, or sink into depression. You may feel cheated by fate or a higher power. But if you don't move beyond this stage, you can become extremely irritable and quarrelsome.

- **Guilt: "I deserved it."** Next, you may blame yourself for having RA. ("I should have been a better person; I should have taken better care of myself," and so on). You may begin to think of yourself as a burden to others. And just as you view your illness as a personal failure, you think if you try harder to do more, you'll feel better.

- **Sadness and depression: "I will miss being able to..."** This stage is a natural part of saying goodbye to lost roles and abilities. It usually gets better in time. However, if this stage persists, depression will set in as a lingering sense of despair and worthlessness. It can also be a quiet cover for anger, anxiety or guilt. Depression persists until negative thinking is changed.

- **Fear and uncertainty: "What else will happen?"** Also natural responses to RA's unpredictable variations, fear and uncertainty themselves may cause muscle tension, increased heart rate, stomach distress, and trembling. Signs that you're stuck in this stage include anticipating the future with fear and anxiety, worrying about the next bad bout even during periods of good health, or feeling helpless or out of control over your health from day to day.

- **Loneliness and isolation: "No one understands."** Curtailing your activities can lead to fewer social contacts. Also, some friends may withdraw because they don't know how to help. Family members may become emotionally exhausted. All these factors can lead to isolation and loneliness if you don't work at broadening your support system and maintaining contact with the outside world.

- **Reconciliation and acceptance: "I may have RA but..."** Acceptance is the final stage of grief, but the first sign you're ready to build a new life. Once you are able to let go of the past and the person you were before you developed RA, you can get on with your recovery.

however, is a severe and prolonged feeling that can hamper your ability to function normally. If you think you may have clinical depression, you should discuss it with a doctor because there are many ways to treat this condition.

Doctors have long debated whether people with rheumatoid arthritis experience higher levels of depression than those without the disease. That's because some signs of depression, such as fatigue and feelings of poor health, are also signs of rheumatoid arthritis. The debate is also related to the issue of a "rheumatoid personality," discussed earlier in this chapter. But most experts do not believe "rheumatoid personality" to be a valid concept. So, many of the questionnaires designed to assess depression in people who have rheumatoid arthritis ask about "physical" rather than "psychological" problems. The answers can then be interpreted to indicate whether a person is depressed.

A second issue is whether depression is more common in women than in men. Women do tend to have higher scores on depression questionnaires, suggesting higher levels of depression. However, one possible explanation is that women are more likely than men to recognize and acknowledge depression, as well as other health problems. It may be that actual

levels of depression are similar in men and women, but a "reporting bias" is picked up by the questionnaire.

Although the debate continues on these issues, some depression associated with the pain, fatigue, uncertainty and loss of function that people who have rheumatoid arthritis face is likely. People fear what may or may not happen as the disease progresses – how arthritis will affect their ability to perform normal activities and to live independently. But depression – like arthritis – is not something to suffer through silently. It can be treated: You can talk to a qualified professional about your feelings, and you can feel better and in more control of your life.

Helplessness

Feelings of helplessness may occur when you are unable to do things you used to do independently or to accomplish as much as you once were able to. As we mentioned in Chapter 18, you can use self-efficacy skills to offset helpless feelings. Studies have shown that people who learn to use self-efficacy skills have improved mental attitudes and physical abilities.

Grief's Parade of Emotions

Grief is a process made up of many feelings, a sort of parade of emotions. In her landmark book *On Death and Dying*, psychiatrist Elisabeth Kübler-Ross, MD, described the stages of grief that terminally ill people go through, and her description has been widely applied to mourning other losses as well. (See the sidebar, "Possible Grief Responses," on page 240.)

However, the stages of grief rarely start at one point and proceed in an orderly way to the ultimate goal of acceptance. For most people, the grief process is more chaotic. You may not experience all the emotions, nor are you likely to experience them step by step. Your reactions may skip around, backtrack or surge together.

Grieving is a personal process that each person goes through at his or her own pace. How you move through the stages of grief depends on your support systems and your basic personality. For example, if you have always been an outgoing person with a sunny disposition, you may not experience the anger or isolation that a more introverted person may feel.

You also need to understand that grief can be ongoing. A worsening of your symptoms, the anniversary of a negative event, or the reminder of an activity that you can no longer do can provoke an unexpected reaction of grief.

Dealing with Grief and Loss

As you consider your losses, use the following tips to help you work through your feelings.

- **Permit yourself to experience your feelings.** Face your loss. Let yourself grieve, cry and be sad. Don't try to ignore anger or punish yourself for feeling it. These emotions are a normal part of the grieving process. As long as they don't last too long, they can help you become more comfortable with the changes in your life. However, if severe depression and crying continue for more than two weeks, see a doctor.

- **Find out what triggers your fears and emotions.** What led to your feelings? What do you need right now that you don't have? If you know you get depressed around certain times of the year, such as an anniversary date, plan to take special care of yourself during that time or plan a special treat for yourself. Avoid situations that create anxiety. This process includes limiting the amount of time you spend around people who make you feel uncomfortable.

- **Express your fears and feelings and then let them go.** Repressing your feelings can be a form of denial, or it can stem from a fear of alienating friends and family. Repressed feelings can fester and grow. Bottling up anger, for example, can

242

Worksheet: Losses and Discoveries List

Use the blanks below to list the losses you've experienced as a result of RA. In the space provided, list the positive things that you may have discovered as a result.

Examples:

Loss: I have lost my independence.
Discovery: I have learned to be comfortable letting other people help.

Loss: I no longer sleep through the night.
Discovery: I feel healthier when I don't drink or eat anything with caffeine. I hardly miss it.

Loss: _____

_____

Discovery: _____

_____

Loss: _____

_____

Discovery: _____

_____

Loss: _____

_____

Discovery: _____

_____

result in excessive irritability, bitterness and quarreling. Repressed feelings also can come out in other destructive ways, such as skipping your prescribed treatment. Some constructive ways of expressing your feelings include talking with others, writing in a journal, crying, screaming in the shower or pounding pillows.

• **Search for meaning.** Draw strength from your spiritual beliefs. Also, think about what positive things have occurred as a result of your rheumatoid arthritis

244

"Grieving the losses in chronic illness has its own peculiar difficulties. You may be struggling with your own grief while also dealing with the mourning of your family. The first time Mother came to visit after my diagnosis, she embraced me and whispered, "Here's some of your grandmother's jewelry. You might as well have it now," and "I'm glad the boys are as old as they are." I ran in stark terror.

"However, the source of the grief process, you, is still present. You are a constant reminder to yourself and others around you of what's been lost.

"After reacting to a diagnosis of chronic illness, your family faces a period of redefinition. In this process, the family's worldview is examined and reformulated. Just as you need to synthesize and incorporate a new identity, your family also needs to adopt one that accepts and understands your new circumstances.

"During this family redefinition, some members' roles will change. You may, for example, always have been responsible for hosting family get-togethers, when you cooked your specialties, polished the silverware and made sure the house gleamed. Now others must help – or even replace – you. In my family, my roles as chief cook , caretaker of my mother, and source of a second income came to a halt as I began to live my life from the bed to the couch to the hospital and back again. Turmoil erupted.

"When it became clear I was seriously ill, everybody in my family pitched in – at first. Later, we hired a maid service to come in once a month to do the heavy house cleaning. The first day the maids came was like a funeral for me, even though I never relished doing housework.

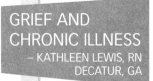

GRIEF AND
CHRONIC ILLNESS
– KATHLEEN LEWIS, RN
DECATUR, GA

"The process of renegotiating and reformulating your new family image is a major transition. Your children or spouse may resent having extra responsibilities. You may resent losing them, along with the identity they gave you as 'provider' or 'homemaker' or 'problem-solver.' But you may find that being 'husband' or 'mother' or 'lover' does not necessarily depend bringing home a fat paycheck or making the perfect puff pastry.

"Life is a highway, and you'll need to pay some tolls. If you try to run them, the consequences could be far more expensive than if you'd thrown your quarters in the basket. In the same way, if you try to put off grief, you may pay a higher price than you will if you face it."

From *Celebrate Life: New Attitudes for Living with Chronic Illness* by Kathleen Lewis, RN
To order this book, call 800-283-7800, or log on to www.arthritis.org.

that might not have happened otherwise. For example you may have:

- reassessed priorities
- discovered inner strengths
- developed new hobbies
- discovered new talents
- made new friends
- increased your understanding of yourself
- increased your understanding of God, a higher power or spirituality, or
- increased your understanding of others with disabilities.

- **Seek professional help when and if you need it.** Often, just talking with an understanding person will be enough to help you through depression or grief. But if you have trouble maintaining your daily activities, feel helpless or hopeless, or have thoughts of hurting yourself or others, seek the guidance of a mental-health professional. See the end of this chapter for help on finding referrals.

Self-Talk

Self-talk is the conversation you have with a voice in your head, and this discussion colors your world view and shapes your expectations. When self-talk is healthy, the voice is a cheering section urging you forward. When it's unhealthy, self-talk holds you back and makes you feel cynical about your life.

Unhealthy self-talk arises from responding automatically to situations with repetitive, negative thinking patterns. These patterns may include a tendency to generalize, to see things in terms of right or wrong and good or bad, to see manageable problems as catastrophes, to place undue significance on only one aspect of an event and to jump to conclusions. Your self-talk is unhealthy when you get stuck on thinking only negative thoughts.

Watch for signs that you may be thinking negatively. Note the way you categorize yourself or others, and the way you judge, label or condemn yourself or others. For example, you may catch yourself saying, "I can't believe what a dumb thing I did," or, "I hate the way I look today." More positive self-talk responses would be "I guess I made a mistake," or "I think I should comb my hair so I will look my best."

Note how often you use words and phrases like *can't, won't, impossible, always, never, should, ought to, must, yes, but* and *if only.* If you constantly use negative terms like these, you may be engaging in unhealthy thinking.

The following are examples of this negative approach to life.

Getting Self-Talk to Work for You

- Write down self-defeating thoughts.

- Do a "Reality Check." Ask:

  - Are there other ways of looking at this situation?

  - What am I afraid will occur?

  - What evidence do I have that this outcome will happen?

  - Is there evidence that contradicts this conclusion?

  - What coping resources are available?

  - Have I only had failures in the past, or were there times I did okay?

  - There are times when I don't do as well as I would like, but other times I do. What are the differences between those times?

- Change self-defeating thoughts to helpful self-talk.

- Mentally rehearse healthy self-talk.

- Practice healthy self-talk in real situations.

- Be patient: it takes time for new patterns of thinking to become automatic.

10 Unhealthy Ways to Think

1. Seeing all or nothing: You place people or situations in black and white categories, with no shades of gray. If your performance falls short of perfect, you see yourself as a total failure.

Healthy response: You recognize an error but place it in the context of all the things you did right.

2. Generalizing: You see a single, unpleasant event as a never-ending pattern of defeat.

Healthy response: You see a single, unpleasant event as a bump in the road.

3. Using mental filters: You pick out a single, unpleasant detail and dwell on it exclusively so that your vision of reality becomes darkened, like the drop of ink that discolors the entire beaker of water.

Healthy response: You pick out the most pleasing detail and dwell on it.

4. Disqualifying the healthy. You reject healthy experiences, such as an acquaintance's remark that you have a great sense of humor, by insisting that it isn't true. In this way you maintain an unhealthy belief such as, "People don't like me," which is contradicted by your everyday experiences.

Healthy response: You embrace healthy experiences such as hearing a compliment about your sense of humor.

5. Jumping to conclusions: You make an unhealthy interpretation even though there are no facts that support your conclusion. Some examples:

a. Mind reading: You conclude that someone is reacting negatively to you and don't find out if you are correct.

b. Fortune telling: You anticipate that things will turn out badly, and you feel convinced that your prediction is an already-established fact.

Healthy response: You assume things are going well (that people like you, that you're doing a good job, etc.) until you learn differently.

6. Magnifying or minimizing: You exaggerate the importance of insignificant events (such as your mistake or someone else's achievement), or you inappropriately shrink the magnitude of significant events until they appear tiny (your own desirable qualities or another person's imperfections). This procedure is also called the "binocular trick."

Healthy response: You celebrate your achievements and others', small and large. If you feel jealous, you acknowledge that and then remind yourself of your own gifts, and share others' happiness.

7. Basing facts on your emotions: You assume that your unhealthy emotions reflect the way things really are: "I feel it, therefore it must be true."

Healthy response: You remind yourself that most days you feel better than you do today.

8. Using "should" statements: You try to motivate yourself with shoulds and shouldn'ts, as if you have to be punished before you can do anything. ("I really should exercise. I shouldn't be so lazy.") Musts and oughts are also offenders. The emotional consequence is guilt. When you direct should statements toward others, you feel anger, frustration and resentment.

Healthy response: You motivate yourself by remembering the good feelings or events that come with the activity. ("Exercise is hard but, boy, I feel good afterward.")

9. Labeling and mislabeling: These are extreme forms of generalizing. Instead of describing your error, you attach an unhealthy label to yourself. You say, "I'm a loser." When someone else's behavior rubs you the wrong way, you attach an unhealthy label to him, such as "He's a real louse." Mislabeling involves describing an event with language that is highly colored and emotionally loaded. Example: Instead of saying someone drops off her children at day care every day, you might say she "abandons her children and lets strangers look after them."

Healthy response: Acknowledge your error, put it in perspective, and move on.

("I'm late to the meeting. That rarely happens. I'll be on time next time.")

10. Personalizing: You see yourself as the cause of some unhealthy external event which in fact you were not responsible for. ("We were late to the dinner party and caused the hostess to overcook the meal. If I had only pushed my husband to leave on time, this wouldn't have happened.")

Healthy response: You do not take on the blame that belongs to other people. ("My husband wouldn't stop watching the basketball game on TV and this made us late to the dinner party. Hey, my husband was rude, but this wasn't my fault.")

Changing Unhealthy Self-Talk

Unhealthy self-talk can make the challenges of rheumatoid arthritis seem like an uphill, impossible battle. Learning to change your self-talk is an important tool in reducing your stress and improving your mood. Here are some ways to make this transformation:

Unhealthy: "I would like to exercise, but I can't. I am also too old to start exercising. I know I can't do it."

Healthy: "Starting an exercise program will give me a chance to get out of the house. I could start slow and easy with a walk in the park or the mall. If I get tired, I can sit down and look at store windows and rest for a while." Or: "Starting an exer-cise program will be a challenge, but I can take it slowly, and it will give me a chance to explore new types of movement."

Unhealthy: "My life will never be the same now that I have RA. I will never be able to do anything that I like to do."

Healthy: "I'm still the same person I've always been. I can cope." Or "I've changed since I was diagnosed with RA, but I'm still a person of worth. I still have a lot to give to people around me."

Unhealthy: "My friends never call me. People don't like being around me."

Healthy: "My friends are just trying to be considerate and spare my energy. They are waiting for signals from me. I'll call today." Or: "My friends are uncomfortable, at a loss, and don't know how to help me. I must ask them for what I need."

Activity: Keep a Thoughts Diary

Paying attention to your thoughts and feelings is the first step in gaining control of unpleasant emotions. During times of emotional turmoil, your thoughts may be so fragmented and jumbled that it's hard to know exactly what they are. Writing in a journal or in a thoughts diary is an excellent way to explore your thoughts and feelings (see the Sample Thoughts Diary below). Because it's your private document, a diary can be a good safety valve for dealing with emotions and stress.

A diary or journal also can flag unhealthy thinking, serve as a reality check and help you process your feelings and thoughts. After you've been writing down your thoughts for a few weeks or months, look back at some of your earlier entries. You may find your perspective has changed.

Avoiding a Spiral Into Depression

Reactions like anger, fear and anxiety are normal parts of the grieving process. They are signals from the body and mind that all is not well and that it is time to mobilize your coping responses. When these emotions are processed by a healthy grieving person, they provide an opportunity to grow and gain new insights. But if they are not dealt with appropriately, they can

Sample Thoughts Diary

To appreciate the power of your self-talk and the part it plays in your emotional life, make your own thoughts diary. Make a notation each time you experience an unpleasant emotion. Include everything you tell yourself to keep the emotion going.

DATE	UNPLEASANT EMOTION	SITUATION	SELF-TALK	RATIONAL RESPONSE
AUGUST 3 9:30 a.m.	depressed, frustrated	In kitchen looking at mess.	I'll never get this kitchen clean.	I'll just do a little bit and get started. No reason to do it all today.
AUGUST 4 10:15 a.m.	tired, discouraged	Putting dishes away.	I should have done a better job of straightening up.	Nothing in the world is perfect, but the room looks better.
AUGUST 6 1:00 p.m.	frustrated	Phone rings and wakes me up from nap.	I should have taken the phone off the hook.	Most days I remember to take the phone off the hook.
AUGUST 7 3:00 p.m.	depressed	Expected call from friend – it didn't come.	I have no real friends. She should have called by now.	Who says she "should" have called me? I think I'll call her.

cause long-term depression. The goal is to process and listen to your feelings, and then release them.

How to Know if You're Depressed

Depression has become a catch-all term. The word sometimes is used inappropriately to refer to brief feelings of sadness or dissatisfaction, what we often call "the blues."

Experiencing a few depressive symptoms every now and then is part of life. But clinical, or major, depression alters the way you view the world and yourself, and may involve changes in the neurotransmitters, or chemicals, in your brain. It may last only several weeks or much longer. And it may interfere with your ability to take pleasure in life, disrupt sleep and cause you to feel helpless and hopeless. Depression can also mask other emotions that are painful to face, like anger or guilt.

It can be hard to recognize depression when you're in the middle of it. Because it can come on gradually, depression can take hold of you before you realize what has happened. Look at the following chart of symptoms to help you determine whether or not you may be experiencing depression.

Remember that RA and some of the medications used to treat it can cause some of the symptoms listed on this chart, particularly low energy and fatigue, changes in appetite and weight, and sleeping too much or too little. So these symptoms alone may not indicate depression. However, you should seek professional help if you have four or more additional symptoms that last for more than two weeks and are severe enough to disrupt your daily life.

If you ever have thoughts of death or suicide, seek professional help immediately. Such thoughts should never be written off as "the blues." Don't let your sad mood become a tragedy. Remember, even the most severe depression is treatable.

Activity: Depression: A Self-Test

Experiencing one or more of these depressive symptoms every now and then is a normal part of life. If a certain number of these symptoms have been bothering you for weeks or years, you may have a depressive disorder and should consult your doctor with this list in hand. See the results below.

Group 1:

Are you experiencing at least one of the following nearly every day?

Apathy, or loss of interest in things you used to enjoy, including sex; sadness; blues; or irritability

Group 2:

In addition, are you experiencing any of the following symptoms?

* Feeling slowed down or restless
* Feeling worthless or guilty
* Changes in appetite or a substantial weight loss or gain
* Problems concentrating, thinking, remembering or making decisions
* Trouble falling asleep or sleeping too much
* Loss of energy, feeling tired all the time

Group 3:

What about the following symptoms? These are not used to diagnose depressive disorders but often occur with them:

* headaches*
* other aches and pains *
* digestive problems*
* sexual problems*
* feeling pessimistic or hopeless
* being anxious or worried
* low self-esteem

Results:

If you have several symptoms, talk to your physician. You may be clinically depressed if you experience at least one of the symptoms in Group 1 and at least four of the symptoms in Group 2 nearly every day for at least two weeks.

Depression Risk Factors

People are at higher risk for depression at certain times in their lives or under certain conditions. You may be at greater risk if:

* You've had a previous episode of depression.

* Your previous depressive episode occurred before age 40.

* You have a medical condition.

* You've just given birth.

* You have little or no social support.

* You've recently experienced a stressful life event (positive or negative).

* You abuse alcohol or drugs.

* You have a family history of depression-related disorders.

* You experienced only partial relief from a previous episode of depression.

Adapted from *Arthritis Today*

You may have chronic depression if you experience at least one of the symptoms in Group 1 and at least two of the symptoms in Group 2 nearly every day for at least two years.

These are potential indications of depression

only if not caused by another disease or by medication.

Reprinted from *Arthritis Today*, January/February 1996.

Seeking Professional Help

If you determine that you are clinically depressed, help is available. Seeing a mental-health professional may have once carried a stigma, but that is no longer the case. Seeing a therapist to help sort out feelings is no different from seeing a dentist for a cavity or a doctor for an infection. A psychiatrist or psychologist (for the distinctions, see Chapter 4) can help you work through your thoughts and emotions by providing an objective, listening ear and offering insight into what you may be feeling or thinking.

Newly developed medications such as SSRIs can address the imbalance of neurotransmitters, or brain chemicals, that may accompany depression. Keep in mind that a psychiatrist is the only mental-health professional who can prescribe medications, although any therapist can refer you to a psychiatrist if medications are necessary.

Even if you're not clinically depressed, you can still benefit from therapy. Dealing with the pain, fatigue and lifestyle changes imposed by RA can be an enormous psychological challenge. Mental or emotional patterns that previously caused minor trouble in your life may now cause major problems. Relationships that functioned satisfactorily without the stress of illness may now call for restructuring and improved communication skills. Or you may simply need a safe place to discuss your feelings. For any of these reasons, therapy might be valuable. You deserve the help you need or want.

Once you have made the decision to seek help from a therapist, how do you go about finding a qualified therapist in your area? If you have health insurance, start by getting a list of therapists your insurance provider will cover. Keep this list with you when you ask your physician or a trustworthy friend or relative to recommend someone. Another way to find a qualified therapist is to call a reputable hospital or mental-health agency in your area.

Today, any number of people call themselves therapists although they have no licenses or training. This practice is not illegal, and some may be good at what they do. But your best bet is to make sure that the person you choose has appropriate mental-health education and training, and belongs to the recognized professional organization for his or her license (for example, the National Association of Social Workers). Often, such an organization will have its own telephone referral line, which will be listed in the telephone directory.

The therapist you find may be a board-certified psychiatrist, licensed clinical psychologist, licensed clinical social worker or licensed marriage, family and child counselor. Therapists who are not

Where To Find Help

The following organizations offer general information on depressive disorders, mental illness, and finding a therapist. Some organizations also have a referral service to help you find a credentialed therapist in your area.

American Association for Marriage and Family Therapy, 112 South Alfred St., Alexandria, VA 22314-3061; 703-838-9808; www.aamft.org

American Psychiatric Association, Department AT, 1000 Wilson Blvd., Suite 1825, Arlington, VA 22209-3901; 703-907-7300; www.psych.org

American Psychological Association, 750 First St., NE, Washington, DC 20002-4242; 800-374-2721; www.apa.org

Depression and Bipolar Support Alliance (DBSA), 730 N. Franklin St., Suite 501, Chicago, IL 60610-7224 ; 800-826-3632; www.dbsalliance.org

Depression Awareness, Recognition and Treatment (D/ART), a program of the National Institute of Mental Health, 5600 Fishers La., Rockville, MD 20857; 800-421-4211; www.brooklane.org

The National Alliance on Mental Illness(NAMI), Colonial Place Three, 2107 Wilson Blvd., Suite 300, Arlington, VA 22201-3042; 703-524-7600; 800-950-NAMI; www.nami.org

National Association of Social Workers, 750 First St., NE, Suite 700, Washington, DC 20002-4241; 202-408-8600; www.naswdc.org

National Foundation for Depressive Illness, P.O. Box 2257, New York, NY 10116; 800-239-1265; www.depression.org.

National Mental Health Association; 201 North Beauregard St., 12th Floor Alexandria, VA 22311; 800-969-NMHA; www.nmha.org

medical doctors, and who thus cannot prescribe drugs, may refer you for psychiatric consultation to evaluate your need for medication.

Once you have obtained some names, don't hesitate to interview a prospective therapist on the phone. Shop around to find a qualified person who makes you feel comfortable. You will discuss personal, emotional and even intimate issues with this person, so you should feel at ease communicating your feelings with any therapist you choose.

Ask about the person's qualifications, training and specific areas of expertise. Ask how much experience the doctor or therapist has had in treating depression. Some therapists have experience treating people with chronic diseases, and it is perfectly appropriate to ask them if they do.

Ask about the fee for services, and make sure you know up front what your insurance will and will not cover. Do you have to pay the fee and wait for full or partial reimbursement from your insurer? You have a right to this information, and a competent professional will not be offended by your questions.

Some therapists are willing to meet with you for an initial session without charge or at a reduced charge, so that you can make an in-person evaluation. Ask the therapist if a free initial consultation is possible.

If you don't have health insurance or if your policy doesn't cover this type of therapy, don't let that stop you from seeking the help you need. Ask your doctor to refer you to community mental-health agencies, which usually use a sliding-fee scale, based on the patient's income, family size and other considerations. Some professionals also may lower their fees, depending on a patient's financial need. And many churches, synagogues and other religious-based institutions offer regular counseling services from clergy who have additional training in therapy or counseling. For information about how and where to find reliable and affordable services, check with your local health or social-services departments.

Chapter 20

Good Living:
Creating a Healthy Lifestyle

We have come a long way in this book, and we've covered quite a bit of information – including information about rheumatoid arthritis, the treatments, and practical suggestions that may help make living with rheumatoid arthritis easier. In fact, you may be feeling overwhelmed by so much information, wondering how you can pull it together into a plan that works for you.

In this chapter, we will try to help you do just that: Take the information that pertains to you and use it to create your own wellness lifestyle. A wellness lifestyle is one in which you are committed to nourishing your body and mind. It includes attitudes and behaviors that help you achieve the highest possible physical, mental and spiritual well-being. Creating a wellness lifestyle is a cornerstone of being a successful self-manager.

Setting Reasonable Goals

Obviously, there are many components to learning to live well with arthritis, or any other chronic disease. And, as we have stressed throughout this book, no two people are alike and no one experiences rheumatoid arthritis in exactly the same way. Take a few moments to look back over the Table of Contents of this book. Some chapters may not apply to you right now. For example, your active disease may be well controlled by medication, so the chapter on surgery may be of less interest to you. Or perhaps you're into exercise and have already worked out what kinds of exercises make you feel better and which ones to avoid.

Now, jot down a few areas you feel you need to change in your life to achieve a wellness lifestyle. The key word here is "few." How many times have you made sweeping New Year's resolutions, only to break them in a couple of weeks and end up feeling guilty and defeated? Changing old habits and creating new ones is hard work. Most experts advise setting reasonable goals that you can live with, rather than trying to change everything in your life at once. An example of a reasonable goal might be something like "I will walk three times a week for 20 minutes," rather than "I will begin training to run the New York marathon."

You may want to make copies of the form below and use them to draw up weekly contracts. This will help you set reasonable goals by listing the specific steps you will take to achieve each goal.

Once you accomplish these goals, you can either raise the bar (for example,

Contract Form

THIS WEEK I WILL: _____ **WEEK OF:** _____

For Example: This week I will <u>walk</u> <u>around the block</u> <u>before lunch</u> <u>three times</u>.
  (WHAT)   (HOW MUCH)   (WHEN)   (HOW MANY)

What

How Much

When

How Many Days

How Certain Are You *(On a scale of 0 to 10 with 0 being totally unsure and 10 being totally confident)*

Signature:

walking 40 minutes instead of 20), or if you've reached a level that you're happy with, you can turn your attention to other areas.

Nourishing Your Mind and Spirit

When you're setting goals, don't forget those that will help you keep a healthy mental, as well as physical, outlook. Taking the time to nourish your mind and spirit can lead to unexpected health benefits like less physical pain, something researchers have found repeatedly to be true for people with chronic diseases.

We aren't always taught how to nourish ourselves emotionally or spiritually. Sometimes, people are taught to do the exact opposite – to ignore their emotions or feelings. However, we can enrich our minds and spirits in many ways, big and small. Consider the following points to help support a healthy mental outlook.

- **Optimism.** Having the view that things in general are pretty good can help you live longer and reduce chronic stress. Expect good things to happen and work toward them. Stop worrying so much. Instead, live one day at a time and use relaxation techniques and healthy self-talk to counter pessimistic thoughts.

- **Humor.** Laughter is good medicine. Author Norman Cousins refers to laughing as internal jogging. Anything that makes you smile brings relief to your mind and spirit. Some research has shown that humor may even improve your immune function.

- **Sense of purpose.** Do you believe you have worth and a purpose for your life and experiences? People who believe in themselves and in the meaning of their lives are happier, more satisfied and serene. This belief in one's self is a choice that occurs regardless of life circumstances.

- **Sense of control.** Do you feel hopeless or frustrated by your arthritis or by other challenges in your life? Given the same situation, some people feel helpless, and others feel a sense of control or confidence that they can influence their own well-being. Goal setting, problem solving, self-monitoring, and communicating your needs and feelings to others are all ways to regain a sense of control.

- **Social support.** Is your life filled with satisfying relationships and love? Do you feel that others understand your arthritis and the demands it places on you? Getting the support you need can be hard work. You need to be a friend to have a friend. You need to be willing to listen to others and communicate your own needs in a clear, direct way.

260

"I wake up to a beautiful spring day. The sun is shining, a warm breeze is blowing, squirrels are playing tag. A rabbit nibbles clover while the blue jay in the pine tree outside my window scolds him. All these things, in addition to walking, I used to take for granted.

"A few years ago, I had routine hip replacement surgery and almost ended up being unable to walk. Several surgeries and thousands of hours of physical therapy later, I'm walking. The length of my walks are still limited; I will never be as strong or as stable was I was before. This can be depressing. When I lose patience and feel like giving up, I talk to a friend who reminds me how far I've come, and how much better I'm doing. Often, I write lists of things I can or cannot do. I compare the recent lists with the old lists. Looking at the improvements I've made, written down on paper, makes them seem more tangible.

SMELLING THE ROSES, WATCHING THE CLOUDS – APPRECIATING LIFE

– SUZIE HERSHMAN, MATAWAN, NJ

"I stop and smell the roses that my husband planted along our driveway. I admire the splendid pinks, reds and oranges in the setting sun. I look out my window while I'm typing and watch the billowy, white clouds float across the sky. Many other wonderful things in my world help me get through the tough days – and the good ones."

Taking Care of the Basics

To live well with rheumatoid arthritis, you should take steps toward healthy living in general. Most of the basics have already been discussed in this book, but they're worth repeating because they are such an important part of feeling healthy and in charge of your life. So keep them in mind as you build your wellness lifestyle:

- **Eat a healthful diet.** Most people with rheumatoid arthritis don't need to follow a special diet. However, you should try to follow the guidelines for a healthy diet described in Chapter 15, in the box on the next page, or explained in the USDA's food pyramid.

- **Get enough sleep.** Many people are sleep deprived due to the demands of work, family and other obligations. We rise early and don't get to bed until late. Lack of sleep increases stress levels and may decrease your body's immune activity. Review the suggestions in Chapter 17 for getting a good night's sleep.

• **Manage stress in healthy ways.** We've talked about ways to reduce stress levels and tips for handling those stresses that can't be eliminated. Resist the temptation to handle stress in unhealthy ways – such as overeating, over-indulging in alcohol or taking drugs – that will only increase stress in the long run.

• **Balance exercise and rest.** Getting regular exercise should be an important part of your wellness lifestyle, but don't forget to balance periods of activity with periods of rest. Taking a 20-minute "breather" may feel like a waste of time, but it may just give you the energy you need to make it through the day.

A Final Word: Making Time for Yourself

Too many people fall into the trap of doing everything that others expect of them but failing to leave enough time for themselves. However, research has shown that your use of time and your overall balance of activities can affect your health and satisfaction with life. Try using the Time Target at the end of this chapter to help you think about how satisfied you are with the amount of time you now spend on activities such as hobbies, time alone or with friends, or other activities that are just for you.

Look for patterns in the Time Target. Is your life balanced so that most or all of the "bull's eye" (the center circle) is colored in? Or do you have a lot of parts of the other circles colored in? Look for colored areas in these outer circles:

• **"Need Less" circle.** If you have a lot of this circle colored in, you may have trouble setting priorities or saying no to others. Are you feeling overwhelmed? If so, go back and read the strategies for dealing with fatigue in Chapter 17 and the effective self-management techniques in Chapter 16.

• **"Need More" circle.** Is it hard for you to ask for what you need? Do you need more from people in relationships? You may need to practice better planning so that you can spend more time on more enjoyable activities. Remember to set goals using a contract, problem solve and plan to create the situation you're after.

• **"Not Important."** If you have colored five or more of the activities as "not important," this may be a sign that you are feeling depressed. If you've lost interest in many activities that you used to enjoy, if you've isolated yourself from friends, or if you feel like hurting yourself, seek professional help. Go back and review the sections on coping with stress and coping with depression in Chapter 19 for additional help.

Finding those things in your life that uplift you and bring you joy and happiness is important. This takes time, patience and determination, but if you can learn to balance each of the hassles in your life with uplifting activities, rheumatoid arthritis can become just a part of your life, not your whole life. Remember: Aim for the bull's eye.

ACTIVITY: Targeting Your Time

Instructions: Read the names for each of the 12 activities listed in the wedges of the circle below. Think about how satisfied you are with the time you now spend on each activity. Color in the part of the wedge for each activity that best describes how that activity fits into your life. For example, if you are satisfied with time spent on an activity, color the center part of the wedge, in the "OK" section. Otherwise, indicate by coloring whether you "need less" or "need more" of the activity, or if the activity is "not important" in your life.

HOW CLOSE ARE YOU TO THE BULL'S-EYE?

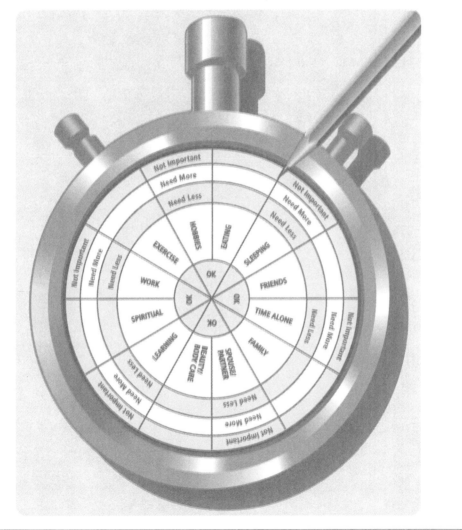

Glossary

acupressure: Eastern medicine technique in which pressure is applied to specific sites along energy pathways called meridians.

acupuncture: Eastern medicine technique in which needles are used to puncture the body at specific sites along energy pathways called meridians.

acute illness: Disease that can be severe, but of short duration, unlike chronic illness.

acute pain: See pain.

adrenal glands: Glands located near the kidneys. These glands secrete a variety of hormones, including glucocorticoids.

adrenaline: A hormone that increases the heart and respiration rate when we feel frightened, threatened or angry, preparing us to flee to safety, or stand and fight.

aerobic: An activity designed to increase oxygen consumption by the body, such as aerobic exercise or aerobic breathing.

alternative therapy: Any practice or substance outside the realm of conventional medicine.

American College of Rheumatology (ACR): An organization that provides a professional, educational, and research forum for rheumatologists across the country. Its functions include helping determine what symptoms and signs define rheumatic disease diagnoses and what the appropriate treatments are for those diagnoses.

analgesic: Drugs used to help relieve pain.

anemia: A condition marked by a reduction in the number of red blood cells, amount of hemoglobin in the blood, or total blood volume.

anemia, iron deficiency: Anemia resulting from a greater demand on the stored iron than can be supplied.

anemia, pernicious: Anemia resulting from a lack of vitamin B12; it is associated with absence of hydrochloric acid in the stomach.

anesthesia: Chemicals that induce a partial or complete loss of sensation. Used to perform surgery and other medical procedures.

anesthesiologist: A physician specializing in the administration of anesthesia.

ankylosing spondylitis: Form of arthritis that primarily affects the joints and ligaments of the spine, marked by pain and stiffness. Can result in fusion of joints and bones, leading to rigidity.

antibody: A specialized protein that neutralizes antigens, or foreign substances, in the body.

antigen: A foreign substance that begins an immune reaction in the body.

antinuclear antibody test: Test used to detect presence of abnormal antibodies.

arthritis: From the Greek word "arth" meaning "joint," and the suffix "itis" meaning "inflammation." It generally means involvement of a joint from any cause, such as infection, trauma or inflammation.

arthrodesis: A surgical procedure involving the fusing of two bones.

arthroplasty: A surgical procedure to replace a joint with an artificial one.

arthroscopic surgery: A type of surgery using an instrument, called an arthroscope, consisting of a thin tube with a light at one end, inserted into the body through a small incision, and connected to a closed-circuit television.

aspiration: The removal of a substance by suction. Technique used to remove fluid from an inflamed joint, both to relieve pressure and to examine the fluid.

autoantibody: antibodies acting against the body's own tissues.

autoimmune disorder: An illness in which the body's immune system mistakenly attacks and damages tissues of the body. There are many types of autoimmune disorders, including arthritis and the rheumatic diseases.

biologic response modifiers: Drugs that target the specific components of the immune system that contribute to disease. Includes etanercept and infliximab.

biomedical model: Traditional model of medical care, based on the principle of identifying a single cause and cure for each disease.

biopsychosocial model: More recent model of medical care, in which a patient's self-management plays a part in the treatment of chronic disease, and biological, psychological and socioeconomic factors are considered influential to the disease's outcome.

body mechanics: The structures and methods with which your body moves and performs physical tasks.

bone densitometry: Imaging study used to measure bone density, particularly in diagnosing osteoporosis.

bunion: Inflammation, enlargement and malalignment of the joint of the great toe.

bursa: A small sac located between a tendon and a bone. The bursae (plural for bursa) reduce friction and provide lubrication. See also bursitis.

bursitis: Inflammation of a bursa (see bursa above), which can occur when the joint has been overused or when the joint has become deformed by arthritis.

Bursitis makes it painful to move or put pressure on the affected joint.

C-reactive protein: Protein that indicates inflammation when found in elevated levels in the body.

capsaicin: A pain-killing chemical contained in some hot peppers, which gives thepeppers their "burn." Available in nonprescription creams that can be rubbed on the skin over a joint to relieve pain.

cartilage: A firm, smooth, rubbery substance that provides a gliding surface for joint motion, and prevents bone-on-bone contact.

chiropodist: a doctor with particular training in the care of the feet. Also called podiatrist.

chronic illness: Disease of a long duration, such as rheumatoid arthritis.

chronic pain: Pain that is constant or persists over a long period , perhaps throughout life. See pain.

circadian rhythm: The daily, monthly and seasonal schedules of essential biologic tasks, such as eating, digesting, eliminating, growing and resting. Disruption of these rhythms – when you travel rapidly across time zones (promoting "jet lag"), for example – has a negative and sometimes profound impact on performance and mood.

complementary therapy: Any practice or substance used in conjunction with traditional treatment.

control group: A group of people used as a standard for comparison in scientific studies.

cool-down exercises: A series of physical activities that allow your heart and respiration rates to return to normal after being elevated by exercise.

corticosteroids: see glucocorticoids.

cortisone: A hormone produced by the cortex of the adrenal gland. Cortisone has potent anti-inflammatory effects but can also have side effects. See also glucocorticoids.

Cox-2 inhibitors: Drugs that inhibit inflammation and are designed to have fewer gastrointestinal side effects than traditional NSAIDs. Includes celecoxib.

cytokines: Chemicals involved in the inflammatory response.

cytotoxic drugs: Chemicals that destroy cells or prevent their multiplication.

deconditioning: Loss of muscle mass and strength because of inactivity. See also reconditioning.

deep breathing: Drawing air into the lungs, filling them as much as possible, and then exhaling slowly. Performing this type of rhythmic breathing for a few minutes increases the amount of oxygen refreshing your brain and produces relaxation and readiness for mental tasks.

depression: A state of mind characterized by gloominess, dejection or sadness.

depression, clinical: A recognized mental illness in which the feelings of depression are severe, prolonged and hamper your ability to function normally.

dermatomyositis: See polymyositis.

disease: Sickness. Some physicians use this term only for conditions in which a structural or functional change in tissues or organs has been identified.

disorder: An ailment; an abnormal health condition.

DMARDs: Disease modifying anti-rheumatic drugs, used to slow or stop the progression of inflammatory joint disease. Includes methotrexate.

dose-pack: A package of glucocorticoid drugs with a tapered daily dosage.

double-blind studies: A method used in scientific studies to compare one intervention (such as a new medication) with other interventions, or no intervention. In this method, the study participants and the persons evaluating the interventions are "blinded" – that is, they aren't told who is getting the intervention being tested – so their responses will not be influenced by their opinions or expectations of the intervention.

endorphins: Natural painkillers produced by the human nervous system that have qualities similar to opiate drugs. Endorphins are released during exercise and when we laugh.

endurance exercises: Exercises such as swimming, walking and cycling that use the large muscles of the body and are dependent on increasing the amount of oxygen that reaches the muscles. These exercises strengthen muscles and increase and maintain physical fitness.

enthesis: The place where the tendon inserts into the bone.

ergonomics: The study of human capabilities and limitations in relation to the work system, machine or task, as well as the study of the physical, psychological and social environment of the worker. Also known as "human engineering."

erosions: Small holes near the ends of bones.

erythrocyte sedimentation rate: A test measuring how fast red blood cells (erythrocytes) fall to the bottom of a test tube, indicating level of inflammation. Often called ESR or "sed rate."

fatigue: A general worn-down feeling of no energy. Fatigue can be caused by excessive physical, mental or emotional

268

exertion, by lack of sleep, and by inflammation or disease.

Felty's syndrome: Form of rheumatoid arthritis marked by an enlargement of the spleen and a reduced number of white blood cells.

fibromyalgia: A noninfectious rheumatic condition affecting the body's soft tissue. Characterized by muscle pain, fatigue and nonrestorative sleep, fibromyalgia produces no abnormal X-ray or laboratory findings. It is often associated with headaches and irritable bowel syndrome.

flare: A term used to describe times when the disease or condition is at its worst.

flexibility exercises: Muscle stretches and other activities designed to maintain flexibility and to prevent stiffness or shortening of ligaments and tendons.

Food Labeling Act: Recent legal decree of the U.S. government mandating the type of information that must be given on food labels regarding nutritional content. This Act ensures that consumers will have easy-to-read fat, protein, fiber, carbohydrate and calorie content information, and more.

gate theory: A theory of how pain signals travel to the brain. According to this theory, pain signals must pass a "pain gate" that can be opened or closed by various positive (e.g., feelings of happiness) or negative (e.g., feelings of sadness) factors.

genetic predisposition: Susceptibility to a specific disease or illness caused by certain inherited characteristics.

glucocorticoids: A group of hormones including cortisol produced by the adrenal glands. They can also be synthetically produced (that is, made in a laboratory) and have powerful anti-inflammatory affects. These are sometimes called corticosteroids or steroids, but they are not the same as the dangerous performance-enhancing drugs that some athletes use to promote strength and endurance.

gout: Disease that occurs due to an excess of uric acid in the blood, causing crystals to deposit in the joint, leading to pain and inflammation.

grief: Feelings of loss; acute sorrow.

guided imagery: A method of managing pain and stress. Following the voice of a "guide," an audiotape or videotape, or one's own internal voice, attention is focused on a series of images that lead one's mind away from the stressor or pain.

H2 blockers: Compounds that act by blocking receptors in the stomach that lead to the production of acid.

hammer toes: A specific type of joint malalignment of the toes seen in rheumatoid arthritis.

helplessness: The concept of not feeling in control of your life or your health.

hematocrit: The percentage of red blood cells found in blood.

hemoglobin: The protein in red blood cells that carries oxygen from the lungs to the tissues.

hormones: Concentrated chemical substances produced in the glands or organs that have specific – and usually multiple – regulating effects on the body.

illness: Poor health; sickness.

immune response: Activation of the body's immune system.

immune system: Your body's complex biochemical system for defending itself against bacteria, viruses, wounds and other injuries. Among the many components of the system are a variety of cells (such as T cells), organs (such as the lymph glands) and chemicals (such as histamine and prostaglandins).

inflammation: A response to injury or infection that involves a sequence of biochemical reactions. Inflammation can be generalized, causing fatigue, fever, and pain or tenderness all over the body. It can also be localized, for example, in joints, where it causes swelling and pain. In rheumatoid arthritis, inflammation is not caused by injury or infection, but is part of an autoimmune reaction.

internist: A physician who specializes in internal medicine; sometimes called a primary-care physician.

isometric exercises: Exercises that build the muscles around joints by tightening the muscles without moving the joints.

isotonic exercises: Exercises that strengthen muscles by moving the joints.

joint: The place or part where one bone connects to another.

joint count: An examination done by a doctor to determine the number of joints that are affected by arthritis.

joint malalignment: When joints are not aligned properly, due to joint damage.

joint replacement surgery: Also known as arthroplasty, a surgical procedure involving the reconstruction or replacement (with a man-made component) of a joint.

ligament: Flexible band of fibrous tissue that connects bones to one another.

locus: The site of a gene on a chromosome.

lupus (systemic lupus erythematosus): The term used to describe an inflammatory connective tissue autoimmune disease that can involve the skin, joints, kidneys, blood and other organs. Associated with antinuclear antibodies.

malalignment, joint: When joints are not aligned properly, due to joint damage.

massage: A technique of applying pressure, friction or vibration to the muscles, by hand or using a massage appliance, to stimulate circulation and produce relaxation and pain relief.

massage therapist: One who has completed a program of study and is licensed to perform massage.

meditation: A sustained period of deep inward thought, reflection and openness to inspiration.

meridians: Energy pathways used in Eastern medicine, but that have no Western medicine counterparts.

morbidity (rate): The frequency or proportion of people with a particular diagnosis or disability in a given population.

MRI: Magnetic Resonance Imaging test, a scan used as a diagnostic aid.

muscle: Tissue that moves organs or parts of the body.

myalgia: Pain of the muscles.

narcotic: A class of drug that reduces pain by blocking signals traveling from the central nervous system to the brain. Although narcotics have the potential to be addictive and are sometimes abused , they can be used safely under skilled medical supervision for effective pain relief.

NSAID (nonsteroidal anti-inflammatory drug): A type of drug that does not contain steroids but is used to relieve pain and reduce inflammation.

nurse: A person who has received education and training in health care, particularly patient care.

nurse practitioner: A registered nurse with advanced training and emphasis in primary care.

objective: Capable of being observed or measured; for example, infection can be objectively observed by the presence of bacteria in a blood test or culture test. See also subjective.

occupational therapist: A health professional who teaches patients to reduce strain on joints while doing everyday activities.

orthopaedic surgeon: A surgeon who specializes in diseases of the bone.

orthopaedist: A physician who specializes in diseases of the bone.

osteoarthritis: A disease causing cartilage breakdown in certain joints (spine, hands, hips, knees) resulting in pain and deformity.

osteoporosis: A disease that causes bones to lose their mass and break easily.

osteotomy: A surgical procedure involving

the cutting of bone, usually performed in cases of severe joint malalignment.

pain: A sensation or perception of hurting, ranging from discomfort to agony, that occurs in response to injury, disease or functional disorder. Pain is your body's alarm system, signaling that something is wrong. Acute pain, stemming from nerve endings stimulated by tissue damage, is temporary and improves with healing. Chronic pain may be mild to severe but persists due to prolonged tissue damage or pain impulses that keep the pain gate open.

palindromic rheumatism: Self-limited attacks of joint inflammation that occur every few weeks or months, then subside after a few days. About one half of people who experience palindromic rheumatism go on to develop chronic rheumatoid arthritis.

pediatrician: A physician with special training who specializes in the diagnosis, treatment and prevention of childhood and adolescent illness.

pediatric rheumatologist: See rheumatologist.

peptic ulcer: A benign (not cancerous) lesion in the stomach or duodenum that may cause pain, nausea, vomiting or bleeding. Such lesions can be caused by nonsteroidal anti-inflammatory drugs such as aspirin or ibuprofen.

pericarditis: Inflammation of the lining surrounding the heart.

pharmacist: A professional licensed to prepare and dispense drugs.

physiatrist: A physician who continues training after medical school and specializes in the field of physical medicine and rehabilitation.

physical therapist: A person who has professional training and is licensed in the practice of physical therapy.

physical therapy: Methods and techniques of rehabilitation that help restore function and prevent disability following injury or disease. Methods may include applications of heat and cold, assistant devices, massage, and an individually tailored program of exercises.

physician: A person who has successfully completed medical school and is licensed to practice medicine.

physician, family: See physician, primary care.

physician, general practitioner: See physician, primary care.

physician, primary care: Physician to whom a family or individual goes initially when ill or for a periodic health check. The physician assumes medical coordination of care with other physicians for the patient with multiple health concerns.

physician's assistant: A person trained, certified and licensed to assist physicians under the supervision by recording medical history and performing the physical examination, diagnosis and treatment of commonly encountered medical problems.

placebo effect: The phenomenon in which a person receiving an inactive drug or therapy experiences a reduction in symptoms.

platelets: Small cells that participate in the formation of blood clotting.

podagra: Gout occurring in the big toe.

podiatrist: A health professional who specializes in care of the foot. Formerly called a chiropodist.

polyarthritis: Arthritis affecting many joints.

polymyositis: Disease in which inflammation occurs primarily in the muscles, leading to muscle weakness and permanent muscle damage. Often associated with dermatomyositis, a condition marked by skin rashes.

PROSORBA Column: Treatment in which certain antibodies associated with rheumatoid arthritis are removed from the blood using a special filtering machine.

proton pump inhibitors: Drugs that block the secretion of acid into the stomach, used to protect the stomach against the gastrointestinal side effects associated with NSAIDs.

psoriatic arthritis: A condition in which psoriasis (a common skin disease) occurs in conjunction with the inflammation of arthritis.

psychiatrist: A physician who trains after medical school in the study, treatment and prevention of mental disorders. A psychiatrist may provide counseling and prescribe medicines and other therapies.

psychologist: A trained professional, usually a PhD rather than an MD, who specializes in the mind and mental processes, especially in relation to human and animal behavior. A psychologist may measure mental abilities and provide counseling.

psychosomatic: Pertaining to the link between the mind (psyche) and the body (soma). pulmonary fibrosis: Scarring of the lungs, leading to shortness of breath.

radiograph: An X-ray.

range of motion (ROM): The distance and angles at which your joints can be moved, extended and rotated in various directions.

Raynaud's phenomenon: Restriction of blood flow to the fingers, toes, or (rarely) to the nose or ears, in response to cold or emotional upset. This results in temporary blanching or paleness of the skin, tingling, numbness and pain.

reconditioning: Restoring or improving muscle tone and strength with appropriate and balanced exercise, nutrition and rest. See also deconditioning.

rehabilitation counselor: A person who guides physical and mental rehabilitation.

relaxation: A state of release from mental or physical stress or tension.

remission: The term used to describe a period when symptoms of a disease or condition improve or even disappear.

remodeling: The regrowth of bone around an artificial joint.

resection: Surgical procedure involving removing all or part of a bone.

resection arthroplasty: A surgical procedure in which resection is done in conjunction with arthroplasty.

revision: A surgical procedure to replace an artificial joint.

rheumatic disease: A general term referring to conditions characterized by pain and stiffness of the joints or muscles. The American College of Rheumatology currently recognizes over 100 rheumatic diseases. The term is often used interchangeably with "arthritis" (meaning joint inflammation), but not all rheumatic diseases affect the joints or involve inflammation.

rheumatoid arthritis: A chronic, inflammatory autoimmune disease in which the body's protective immune system turns on the body and attacks the joints, causing pain, swelling and deformity.

rheumatoid factor: An abnormal antibody often found in blood of people with rheumatoid arthritis.

rheumatoid nodules: Lumps of tissue that form under the skin, often over bony areas exposed to pressure, such as on the fingers or around the elbow.

rheumatologist: A physician who pursues additional training after medical school and specializes in the diagnosis, treatment and prevention of arthritis and other rheumatic disorders.

rheumatologist, pediatric: A rheumatologist who specializes in the diagnosis, treatment, and prevention of arthritis or other rheumatic diseases in children and adolescents.

salicylates: A subcategory of NSAIDs, including aspirin.

scleritis: Inflammation of the eyes.

scleroderma: A connective tissue disease characterized by a tightening of the skin, and a discoloration of the hands when exposed to cold (known as

Raynaud's phenomenon). Can affect internal organs as well.

scleromalacia perforans: Permanent eye damage caused by severe inflammation

self-efficacy: The concept of a person having emotional control in reaction to events in their life, such as a chronic illness.

self-help: Any course, activity, or action that you do for yourself to improve your circumstances or ability to cope with a situation.

self-management: The concept of a person having control of his or her disease and its management.

self-talk: The voice in your head that you use to talk to yourself, aloud or in thought.

shared epitope: Genetic marker that approximately two-thirds of people with rheumatoid arthritis have.

Sjögren's syndrome: Syndrome affecting the salivary and lacrimal (tear-producing) glands, leading to dry eyes and dry mouth.

skeletal muscles: The voluntary muscles that are involved primarily in moving parts of the body. "Voluntary" in this sense refers to muscles that move in response to our decisions to walk, bend, grasp, and so on, as opposed to muscles such as the heart, which do their work without our willful direction.

social worker: A person who has professional training and is licensed to assist people in need by helping them capitalize on their own resources and connecting them with social services (for example, home nursing care or vocational rehabilitation).

soft-tissue rheumatism: Pertaining to the many rheumatic conditions affecting the soft (as opposed to the hard or bony) tissues of the body. Fibromyalgia is one type of soft-tissue rheumatism. Others are bursitis, tendinitis and focal myofascial pain.

spontaneous remission: A somewhat rare disappearance of symptoms of rheumatoid arthritis, usually occurring in the early stage of disease.

steroids: A group name for lipids (fat substances) produced in the body and sharing a type of chemical structure. Among these are bile acids, cholesterol, and some hormones. Not the same as anabolic steroids, drugs synthesized from testosterone (the male sex hormone) and used by some athletes to promote strength and endurance.

strain: Injury to a muscle, tendon or ligament by repetitive use, trauma or excessive stretching.

strengthening exercises: Exercises that help maintain or increase muscle strength.

See also isometric exercises and isotonic exercises.

stress: The body's physical, mental and chemical reactions to frightening, exciting, dangerous or irritating circumstances.

stressor: Factors that cause stress in your life.

symmetric arthritis: Arthritis affecting the same joints on both sides of the body.

syndrome: A collection of symptoms and/or physical findings that characterize a particular abnormal condition or illness.

synovectomy: Surgical removal of the synovium, or the lining of the joint.

synovitis: Inflammation of the lining of the joint.

synovium: The lining of the joint.

synovial fluid: The fluid found in the joint.

systemic disease: A disease that may affect more than one system in the body.

target heart rate: The number of heartbeats per minute to reach during exercise in order to gain maximum benefits. Because the normal heart rate changes as we age, target heart rates are grouped by age.

tendinitis: Inflammation of a tendon.

tendon: A cord of dense, fibrous tissue uniting a muscle to a bone.

TENS: a treatment for pain involving a small device that directs mild electric pulses to nerves in the painful area.

teratogenic: Causing the malformation of a fetus.

thrombocytopenia: Decreased number of platelets.

tissue: A collection of similar cells that act together to perform a specific function in the body. The primary tissues are epithelial (skin), connective (ligaments and tendons), bone, muscle and nerves.

titer: A standard of strength per volume or units per volume.

trochanteric bursitis: Irritation of the trochanteric bursa, which is located on the bony prominence of the femur or thigh. See also bursitis.

Type I disease: Term used to describe rheumatoid arthritis that meets certain criteria, including symptoms that do not last long or progress in severity.

Type II disease: Term used to describe rheumatoid arthritis that meets certain criteria including inflammation in symmetrical joints for longer than six months, and no spontaneous remission of symptoms. A mild disease course that can be controlled with less aggressive therapy.

Type III disease: Most severe form of rheumatoid arthritis, with greater severity of symptoms than Type II disease, requiring aggressive therapy.

uric acid: Substance formed when the
body breaks down waste products
called purines. Uric acid crystals
deposited in the joints cause gout.

urinalysis: Test done on the urine to
detect levels of sugar, protein or
abnormal cells.

vasculitis: Inflammation of the blood vessels.

visual analogue scale: A tool used to measure subjective feelings such as pain on
a scale of 0 to 10 or 0 to 100.

visualization: A method of imaginative
thinking that allows you to picture
achieving – and perhaps achieve – a
goal.

warm-up: Gentle movement to warm up
the muscles before performing
stretches and more strenuous exercise.

Index

A

Abatacept, 116, 117, 120, 133

Acceptance, as grief response, 240

Acetaminophen, 96, 103ñ104, 131

    with codeine, 131

Activity, balancing rest and, 203-204

Actron, 129

Acupuncture/acupressure, 149-150, 197, 265

Acute disease, 265

    versus chronic disease, 83ñ84

Adalimumab, 116, 117, 119-120, 133

Adrenal glands, 20, 265

    effect of long-term use of corticosteroids
      on, 109

Adrenaline, 265

Advil, 96, 97, 99, 129

Aerobic exercises, 169-171, 265

Aggressive therapy. See Drugs

Aging, 217

Aids for Arthritis, Inc., 207

Alcohol, drinking, in moderation, 188-189

Aleve, 96, 97, 99-100, 130

All You Need to Know About
    Joint Surgery, 138

Alternative therapies, 147-159, 265

acupuncture/acupressure, 149-150, 197

    cautions in trying, 157

    diet or dietary changes, 150-151

    exercise, 148, 163-183, 197

    getting more information on, 148

    guided imagery, 148, 202, 233-237

    herbs, supplements and natural remedies,
      152-158

    making smart choices about, 159

    massage, 148-149, 197

    prayer and spirituality, 158

    relaxation, 148, 197, 202, 229-230,
      231-233

    talking to doctor about, 158-159

Alternative Treatments for Arthritis:
    An A to Z Guide, 148, 158

American Association for Marriage and
    Family Therapy, 253

American Cancer Society, 151

American College of Rheumatology (ACR),
    103, 265

American Heart Association, 151, 186-187,
    188

American Psychiatric Association, 253

American Psychological Association, 253

Americans with Disabilities Act (ADA), 64

Anacin, 128, 131

Anaflex 750, 130

Anakinra, 116, 119, 133

Analgesics, 102-106, 131, 265

acetaminophen, 96, 103-104, 131

    narcotic, 104-106

Anaprox, 130

Anemia, 34, 81, 212-213, 265

Back kick (hip extension), 180

Bargaining, as grief response, 240

Baseline X-rays, 79

Bayer, 96, 128

Behavioral medicine, 158

Bextra, 102

Bicycling, 170

Biologic response modifiers, 86, 113,
116-121, 133, 266
abatacept, 116, 120
adalimumab, 116, 119-120
anakinra, 116, 119
etanercept, 116, 117-118
infliximab, 116, 118
rituximab, 116, 120-121

Biomedical model, 7-8, 266

Biopsychosocial model, 7, 266
for arthritis care, 7-12, 62

Black currant oils, 155

Blood, components of, 34

Blood cells, effects of methotrexate on
formation of, 114

Blood clots, 142

Blood counts, 80-81

Blood-forming cells, rheumatoid
arthritis and, 55

Blood serum, 35

Blood urea nitrogen (BUN), 54

B-lymphocytes, 17, 35, 116, 120

Body, rhythms of, 215

Body mechanics, 203, 266

Bone densitometry, 39, 266

Bone remodeling, 139-140

Bone scans, 38-39

Borage oils, 155

Boron, 155

Boswellian, 155

Bufferin, 96, 128

Bunions, 266

Bursa, 45-46, 266

Bursitis, 4, 5, 45-46, 100, 110, 266-267

Button test, 29

C

Calf stretch, 182

Capsaicin, 155, 267

Carbohydrates, 187-188
complex, 188
simple, 187-188

Cardiovascular (aerobic) exercises, 169-171

Carpal tunnel syndrome, 110

Cartilage, 21, 267

Cataflam, 128

Cat's claw, 155

Cayenne, 155

CD20-positive, 120

Celebrex, 97, 102, 131

Celecoxib, 97, 102, 131

Cementless joints, 139-140

Cemeted joints, 139-140

Chemotherapy, 111

Chest stretch, 183

Children, arthritis in, 3-4

Chin tucks, 173

Chiropodists, 72, 267

Chloroquine, 111, 122

Grip strength, 29

Guided imagery, 148, 202, 233-237, 269

Guilt, as grief response, 240

H

H2 blockers, 101, 269

combining NSAIDs with, 101

Hair loss, methotrexate as cause of, 115-116

Hammer toes, 270

Head tilts, 174

Head turns (rotation), 173

Health Assessment Questionnaire (HAQ), 27

Health-care team, 10-11, 69-75

doctors on, 70-72

getting the most from, 73-74

members of, 69-70

nurse practitioners on, 72

nurses on, 72

occupational therapists on, 73

pharmacists on, 73

physical therapists on, 73

physician assistants on, 73

rehabilitation counselors on, 73

social workers on, 73

Taking P.A.R.T. method, 74-75

Heart, rheumatoid arthritis and, 54

Heart rate ranges, recommended, 171

Heat therapy, 197, 199, 201-202

Helplessness, 195, 224-225, 241, 270

Hematocrit, 34, 270

Hemoglobin, 34, 270

Herbs, 152-158

Hexadrol, 132

Hip abduction/adduction, 180

Hip extension, 180, 183

Hip internal/external rotation, 181

Hip/knee flexion, 179

Hip replacement, rehabilitation after, 143-144

Hip turns, 181

HLA-B27, 45

HLA shared epitope, 19-20

Honey, 188

Hormone replacement therapy, 217

Hormones, 270

Human lymphocyte antigen (HLA), 19

Humira, 116, 119, 133

Humor, sense of, 197

Hydrocodone, 104

Hydrocortisone, 132

Hydrocortone, 132

Hydroxychloroquine, 110, 111, 114, 121, 122-123

Hydroxychloroquine sulfate, 135

Hyperadrenocorticism, 107

I

Ibuprofen, 34, 96, 97, 99, 129

Illinois Assistive Technology Program, 206

Illness, 270. See also Disease

Imaging studies, 38-39, 79

bone densitometry, 39

bone scans, 38-39

joint ultrasound, 39, 79

magnetic resonance imaging (MRI), 39, 79

radiographs (X-rays), 16, 38, 62, 79

Immune complexes, 17

289

Natural remedies, 152-158

Neck exercises, 173

Neoral, 54, 122, 134

Neurological disorders, 120

Nexium, 101

Nizatidine, 101

Non-Hodgkin's lymphona, 55, 120

Nonsteroidal anti-inflammatory drugs
(NSAIDs), 34, 54, 59, 81, 86, 96,
97-101, 128-130, 142, 153, 271
aspirin as classic, 98
gastrointestinal irritation and, 98, 100-101
traditional, 99-100

North Coast Medical, 207

Nuprin, 99, 129

Nurse(s), 72, 271

Nurse practitioners, 72, 271

Nutrition. See also Diet
poor, 151

Nutrition resources, 190

O

Oat bran, 188

Objective, 271

Occupational therapists, 73, 186, 271

Omega-3 fatty acids, 153

Omepraxzole, 101

On Death and Dying (K¸bler-Ross), 242

Ophthalmologists, 52

Optic neuritis, 117, 120

Oral gold, 111, 124, 134

Oral ulcers, 52, 116

Orasone, 132

Orencia, 116, 120, 133

Orthopaedic surgeons, 71-72, 138, 143, 271

Orthopaedists, 3, 71-72, 271

Orudis, 100, 129

Orudis-KT, 96, 129

Oruvail, 100, 129

Osteoarthritis, 4, 5, 41-43, 100, 104, 271
distinguishing between rheumatoid
arthritis and, 43
erosive, 42

Osteoporosis, 39, 271

Osteotomy, 141, 271-272

Over-the-counter drugs versus prescription
drugs, 85-87

Overuse, 172

Oxaprozin, 100, 130

Oxycodone, 104

P

Pain, 272
chronic, 198
cycle of, 224-225
defined, 196
exercise and, 171-172
experience of, in head, 103
gate theory of, 196-198
in joints, 26-27
managing chronic, 202-203
relaxation, in controlling, 231-233
symmetric, 26

Pain management, 6-7, 195-207
avoiding joint pain and damage, 203-204
for chronic pain, 202-203

V

Valdecoxib, 102

Vasculitis, 5, 48, 52, 277

Vegetables, 187-188

Vicodin, 103

Vioxx, 102

Vision impairments, hydroxychloroquine
and, 122

Visual analogue scale, 196, 277

Visualization, 277

Voltaren, 100, 101, 128

Voltaren XR, 128

W

Walking time, 29, 170

Walk With Ease, 295

Warm-up, 277

Water exercise, 170

Weight, surgery and, 142

White blood cells, 17, 19, 34, 35

White cell count, 34

Whole grains, 187-188

Willow bark, 157-158

Work disability, 62-64

Wrist bend (extension), 177

Wrist exercises, 177

Wygesic, 131

X

X-rays, 16, 38, 79
changes in joint damage in, 62

Z

Zantac, 101

Zero-order release aspirin, 97, 98

Zinc sulfate, 158

Zingiber offinale, 156

ZORprin, 98, 128

Resources for Good Living

The Arthritis Foundation, the only national, voluntary health organization that works for the more than 66 million Americans with arthritis or chronic joint symptoms, offers many valuable resources through more than 150 offices nationwide. Your local chapter has information, products, classes and other services to help you take control of your arthritis or related condition. To find the chapter office nearest you, call 800-568-4045 or search the Arthritis Foundation Web site at www.arthritis.org.

Programs and Services

• Physician referral – Most Arthritis Foundation chapters can provide a list of doctors in your area who specialize in the evaluation and treatment of arthritis and arthritis-related diseases.

• Exercise programs – The Arthritis Foundation sponsors, develops and coordinates exercise programs for people with arthritis, featuring specially-trained instructors. They include:

    1) *Walk With Ease* – This course allows participants to develop a walking plan that meets their individual needs, accompanied by the Arthritis Foundation book *Walk With Ease: Your Guide to Walking for Better Health, Improved Fitness and Less Pain.* A new audio walking guide is now available to use during your walking routines, with guidelines, upbeat music and inspiring motivation. In addition, a Walk With Ease group leader's manual is available to help you start and lead a walking group in your area.

    2) *Arthritis Foundation Exercise Program* – Relieve stiffness and lessen arthritis pain by doing low-impact exercises designed for people with arthritis and taught by trained instructors.

    3) *Arthritis Foundation Aquatic Program* – Join in the fun of a six- to 10-week exercise program in an heated pool led by trained instructors.

    4) *Arthritis Foundation Self-Help Program* – Learn how to take control of your own care in this six-week class for people with arthritis. This program was developed at Stanford University.

Information and Products

Find the latest information about arthritis, including research, medications, government advocacy, programs and services through one of the many information resources offered by the Arthritis Foundation:

• www.arthritis.org – Information about arthritis is available 24 hours a day on the

Internet at the Arthritis Foundation's interactive, comprehensive Web site. Find news about arthritis, ways to get involved, and a variety of useful arthritis products, including books, brochures, videos and more.

- Arthritis Answers – Call toll-free at 800-568-4045 for 24-hour, automated information about arthritis and Arthritis Foundation resources. Trained volunteers and staff are also available at your local Arthritis Foundation chapter to answer questions or refer you to physicians and other resources. Or e-mail questions to help@arthritis.org.

- Books – The Arthritis Foundation publishes a variety of books on arthritis to help you learn to understand and manage your condition, live a healthier life, and cope with the emotional challenges that come with a chronic illness. Order books directly at www.arthritis.org or by calling 800-283-7800. All Arthritis Foundation books are available at your local bookstore.

- Brochures – The Arthritis Foundation offers brochures containing concise, understandable information on the many arthritis-related diseases and conditions. Topics include surgery, the latest medications, guidance for working with your doctors and self-managing your illness. Single copies are available free of charge at www.arthritis.org or by calling 800-568-4045.

- *Arthritis Today* – This award-winning bimonthly magazine provides the latest information on research, new treatments, trends and tips from experts and readers to help you manage arthritis. A one-year subscription to Arthritis Today is included when you become a member of the Arthritis Foundation. Annual membership is $20 and helps fund research to find cures for arthritis. Call 800-283-7800 for information.

- *Kids Get Arthritis Too* – This newsletter focusing on juvenile rheumatic diseases, is published six times a year. Features speak to children and teens with the illness as well as to their parents. Stories examine the latest news in diagnosis, treatment and research of children's rheumatic diseases, as well as helpful ways kids can cope with their illnesses and the challenges they bring. This newsletter is free. To sign up, e-mail kgatmail@arthritis.org or write *Kids Get Arthritis Too*, 1330 West Peachtree Street, NW, Suite 100, Atlanta, GA 30309.

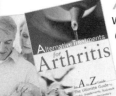